Finally Free

Breaking the Bonds of Depression
Without Drugs

Patty Mason

Endorsements

"Anyone who has experienced depression knows that hope is oxygen. This book is an air hose. Patty Mason has courageously pulled back the curtain on her frightening experience of depression, so we may know we are not alone. With honesty, she describes the descent of despair, and with gentleness escorts us on the journey of not just her own recovery, but ours as well. Patty also offers wise guidance to those seeking to support a depressed loved one. *Finally Free* will encourage and help a LOT of people. It will literally save some people's lives."

– **Ramon Presson**, Ph.D., M.S.
Clinical Therapist, Columnist,
Author of *When Will My Life Not Suck?: Authentic Hope for the Disillusioned*

"*Finally Free* is interesting, compelling and encouraging. I'm always interested in reading about how God works in a person's life. Patty needed God, and God found her and freed her from depression. Her story, though, is about more than depression. The bigger story is about how God restored her soul in numerous ways, reassuring us that whatever our problem is, God wants to help us. If you need help believing this, read Patty's story and be encouraged."

– **Brenda Poinsett**, author of *30 Days of Hope for Dealing with Depression and When Saints Sing the Blues: Understanding Depression through the Lives of Job, Naomi, Paul and Others*

"Hope. That's exactly what our world needs and is constantly seeking. One of the greatest ways to share hope is to share from our own experience how we have not only survived the trials, but thrived. In *Finally Free*, Patty shares her story of how God delivered her from the pit of depression to offer the reader hope that they too can be finally free."

– **Dr. Michelle Bengtson**, neuropsychologist, Author
of *Hope Prevails: Insights from a
Doctor's Personal Journey Through
Depression and Hope Prevails Bible Study*

"Could not put this book down! Patty's story is so familiar to anyone who has battled depression, either personally or with a family member. Yet it is very unique because of her hope and joy. Patty will give YOU hope in your darkest hour, and will help you to live the way God intended, abundantly, and with joy and enthusiasm."

– **Dr. Mike and Doris Courtney**,
Founder of Branches Counseling Center,
Author of *Failure and How I Achieved It*

"If you suffer from depression or know someone who does, you will want to read *Finally Free: Breaking the Bonds of Depression Without Drugs*. Patty Mason shares her story in a raw and vulnerable way that immediately connects her to the reader. Patty has experienced God's healing, grace, and love from being open and honest with him, and admitting her desperate need for a Savior. You will definitely feel encouraged and hopeful that God wants that same freedom for you."

– **Deanna Fullerton**, MA, Licensed
Clinical Pastoral Counselor

"Loved *Finally Free*, its honesty and transparency. This book has been a blessing and revealed things I need to work on. It reminded me to receive God's love in areas of brokenness."

— **Marianne Lynch**

"In *Finally Free*, Patty Mason reveals her failed attempt to climb out of depression and God's miraculous intervention that set her free and brought her joy and purpose. Her gentle spirit and personal experience, both as a victim and a caregiver, offer hope and practical help to those facing this oppressive giant."

— **Debbie W. Wilson**, Biblical Counselor, Life Coach, Author of *Little Women, Big God* and *Give Yourself a Break*

"If there were any doubt God performs modern day miracles, Patty takes away that doubt with her complete transparency in her story of abuse, depression, and healing. As the story unfolded, tears streamed down my face. I felt as if I traveled this journey right along with her. "Living" her miracle moment made me re-live mine. I know EXACTLY what she was feeling!"

— **Celeste Vaughn**

"Patty Mason shares genuinely and openly about her struggle with depression, and her victory in overcoming it. What a testimony of courage, strength, authenticity and faith. Depression strikes many, but Patty shows the way to discover individual freedom. This book is a friendly voice in the fog, a light in the darkness, and truth to dispel the stereotype."

— **Jennifer Johnson**

"A compelling memoir with straightforward direction in drop-kicking depression without drugs. *Finally Free* is worth reading to gain insight from one who broke the bonds. This compelling story moves the reader along. Impactful statements throughout the book awaken the reader with inspirational insight and motivational actions to be victorious on the battlefield of depression."

– Carolyn Knefely, Teacup Ministries,
co-founder of Christian Communicators

"Patty's own healing from depression sets the tone for this encouraging book. She knows, firsthand, how God can shine his light into a life consumed by darkness. Today Patty is an enthusiastic woman who speaks out about depression. Her new life after depression is loaded with joy and purpose. I feel the passion of Patty's words. She truly knows there is hope, and through this book she wants to help others find freedom from depression. She is living proof that with God all things are possible."

– Maxine Marsolini, Founder
of Rebuilding Families

"*Finally Free* offers a beautiful blend of gripping details, moving episodes, and important facts. With fresh candor, the author reveals intimate scenarios that stir in the reader a desire to know more. *Finally Free* is an anointed resource. A must-read for those who desire to leave the dark valley of depression and walk onto the freedom that Christ's miraculous love offers."

– Janet Perez Eckles, International Speaker, Author,
and Founder of
JC Empowerment Ministries

**Finally Free: Breaking the Bonds
of Depression Without Drugs**

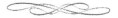

For Angie, and all those who are suffering, or who have suffered, with depression. You always have hope.

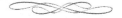

Table of Content

Introduction

Before We Begin...

You need to know you are not alone in the battle. Depression is the number one leading cause of disability worldwide. In a recent report, the Anxiety and Depression Association of America states that "an estimated 40 million American adults, age eighteen or older, experience depression each year,"[1] and that number continues to grow. Depression is a crushing illness that pays no attention to age, nationality, gender, social status, or skin color. "Women are especially at risk—one in eight women develop depression at some point during their lifetime."[2]

Yet in spite of these overwhelming statistics, you also need to know there is hope. You may not feel hopeful. I understand. I too was in a pit of depression. I couldn't see any way out and believed the darkness would never end. If you suffer from depression, I know the pain you face every day. I know you are hurting emotionally, spiritually, and physically. I know the sense of hopelessness and despair. I understand the isolation and feelings of abandonment by others, even by those you once called friend. I know you long to end the madness and stop feeling like a prisoner in your own skin. I know you ache to escape the emotional turmoil consuming and destroying your life. I understand because I've been there. Yet in the midst of my nightmare, I found freedom. I found a way out of that well. And now that I'm on the other side of depression, I'm here to tell you there is an answer. There is a way to be *finally free.*

Throughout this book, I'll let you into my battle with depression, the struggles I faced, and the depth of despair that drove me to thoughts of suicide. Yet through my story, my greatest desire is to offer hope to those suffering with depression, as well as those living with a depressed loved one.

Many things can cause depression. Major or clinical depression can be brought on by a chemical inconsistency in the brain, such as persistent depressive disorder or bipolar disorder, and can even be passed down genetically.

Women can experience depression due to hormonal imbalance. For example, many mothers experience what is known as the "baby blues" due to hormonal changes, lack of sleep, and the pressures of taking care of a new baby. But 10-to-15 percent of these new mothers can experience what is called "postpartum depression," lasting from one month to a year after the baby is born.

Depression can be seasonal. Certain holidays, or certain times of the year, can bring on feelings of despair. Trauma affects the brain, so life-altering events, such as the loss of a loved one, abandonment, abuse, or a tragic accident can cause depression. Loss of employment, chronic illness, obesity, loneliness, addiction, or deep financial debt can trigger depression. Repressed or unhealthy emotions, such as anger, bitterness, envy, comparison, unforgiveness, fear, worry, anxiety, disappointment and discouragement, can generate depression. Any harmful emotion we allow to fester and take root in our heart can be a basis for depression. Sin and rebellion can cause depression. We can even produce feelings of depression by dwelling on negative thought patterns, such as constantly thinking and speaking destructive or harmful words to ourselves. Poor diet or lack of sleep and exercise can also play a factor in depression and its level of severity. Yet regardless of how or why the depression surfaced, it's important to hold on to the truth that there is hope.

In an effort to feel better, many will turn to doctors and medication for relief. I did. However, although I sought a prescription treatment, I never went on medication. Medication was *not* the answer to my problems.

Understand that not all depression requires medication. Plus, taking anti-depressants comes with the risk of physical side-effects and can cause other mental health issues. Depending on your condition and type of depression, counseling, therapy, or medical treatment may be an option. But medication was not what helped me get out of that well. That's not my story of how I became *finally free*.

As you read my story, if you are struggling yourself, my hope is you will discover renewed strength, courage, and determination—and your soul will find healing and freedom from emotional pain. If you are living with someone who is suffering, I pray my story will give you insight into the challenge, darkness, and pain your loved one is facing. If you have not experienced depression yourself, it is difficult to understand what a depressed person is going through. In the *Special Addition* section of this book, I offer some practical tips and tools to help you as a caregiver.

Whatever side of the well you may be on, allow my experience to inspire you to move forward and get to the root of the depression. And permit my story to comfort you in the midst of the suffering and bring you renewed hope.

With love,

Patty

CHAPTER 1

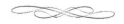

The Trouble with Depression

I Never Saw It Coming

To know me today you would never guess I battled depression; a prisoner who lived within the dark walls of torment, enslaved by despair and the fury of pent-up rage. You would never guess I lived through a darkness so blinding, a pain so unbearable, and an isolation so devastating, I became suicidal.

What is it about depression that brings a seemingly normal, sane woman to the brink of wanting to take her own life? What is it about depression that drives a soul to want to forsake her own existence and see death as an option for escape?

For those who have never experienced this devastating condition, this may be an inconceivable and illogical concept that is unreasonable. You may even feel frustrated and wonder why people don't just get over it. At least that's what my husband thought. It wasn't because he didn't care. At the time, he didn't understand why I couldn't shake it off—to make the *choice* to be happy. But depression is not some temporary mood you wake up from and get over. People who have never experienced depression do not understand the difficult struggle we face every day.

Depression was a constant battle bringing on overwhelming feelings of sadness, rage, and hopelessness. I felt alone and lost—nothing mattered anymore. Feelings of guilt and worthlessness plagued my mind. I became restless, easily flustered and had trouble concentrating. I was in a miserable place, and it didn't take long to have thoughts of death and suicide invade my mind.

Depression devastated, debilitated, and demoralized my life. It crippled my mind, heart, spirit, and soul and destroyed every part of me. Nothing bound me in a world of pain and suffering like depression. It captured me and refused to let go. It was an unceasing vacuum that gripped my soul in such a way that it rendered me utterly helpless and hopeless. I couldn't control what was happening. My once energetic personality lost its drive. I felt drained and tired, and lost all interest to do anything or go anywhere.

When the symptoms appeared, I felt confused and wondered why I felt this way. *Where did I go wrong?* At the time, I was living a good life—a life that appeared to be full of hopes and dreams, plans and expectations that kept me hungering for more. So what happened? How could the highest point of my life so quickly become the lowest? It made no sense, but when the depression surfaced, my world crashed, and I didn't have the faintest idea how to pick up the pieces, much less put them back together.

I never saw the depression coming, nor did I realize how much it would steal from me. Nonetheless, depression hit my life like a freight train going about ninety miles an hour. I didn't expect it or plan for it; yet there it was, like an unwelcome guest in my home.

The truth of the matter is no one ever sees depression coming into their life. They do not forecast it, nor plan for it. Depression is not a lifelong aspiration. No one asks for it, desires it, deserves it, or relishes in the fact they have it. No one ever sets out to be depressed. It's a condition that often appears without warning, like a dark storm that appears on the horizon of a sunny day, and destroys everything in its path.

The Story Begins...

I would say my battle with depression unknowingly began at the age of eighteen, on the day I decided to *find* myself. The symptoms didn't surface at the age of eighteen. They appeared years later, when I was thirty-five. Depression has a root. In order to fully appreciate my story, you need to know its origin and how it brought me to a point of despair. No depression story begins when the symptoms become visible. From my perspective, depression took root when I went down the paths I thought would bring me a sense of worth and fulfillment.

This may seem odd. After all, how could a quest for fulfillment bring me, or anyone, to depths of despair? It's puzzling, but to see that it's possible, all we have to do is watch the news to learn of another outwardly successful life that was cut short.

A doctor would likely say the depression took root much earlier, probably during my childhood and teen years. Deep feelings of anger certainly took root then. I suffered a great deal of physical and emotional abuse. My father didn't understand love, and took a military and corporal approach to discipline. He didn't know any other way to rear his children, so he passed along the only method of discipline he knew and understood.

I grew up in a state of continual fear. My mother, on the other hand, was the exact opposite. Overcompensating for my father's strict physical discipline, she offered no discipline at all. It was two extremes attempting to find a middle ground, both convinced their way of doing things was correct.

School was no refuge either. As a timid child full of fear and insecurity, I became the outcast, the brunt of everyone's cruel jokes, and a constant object of teasing and harassment.

One recess in particular, when I was in sixth grade, a group of kids—both boys and girls—taunted me until they trapped me in a corner against a brick wall. Once they realized I couldn't escape, they began to hurl snowballs filled with rocks at my head and face. This went on until the school bell rang calling us back to class. No one saw, no one stopped the attack, and no one asked any questions. It was a mortifying incident I never forgot.

My family moved a great deal when I was young, and each time we moved I knew what was coming. Although I hoped every new location would offer a chance to start over and leave the former things behind, it was always the same. The kids were the same, the mean jokes were the same, life in general was the same. Over time, my humiliation grew to resentment, anger, and bitterness, that festered beneath the old feelings of fear, insecurity, and loneliness.

When I turned thirteen, those suppressed emotions surfaced and manifested for the first time, and I started lashing out at everyone around me, even those I loved. In what seemed like a flash, I went from

a sweet, shy, soft-spoken child to an a'
full of rage and resentment. I screamed
and threw temper tantrums. No longer able
years of fear, hurt, and abuse, my teen years were in
raging water continually bursting through the dam of
my broken heart.

By the time I turned eighteen, I didn't realize the
effects those childhood events had, and would have,
on my soul. I didn't recognize the emotional wounds I
had buried. I didn't understand how a series of events,
coupled with my anger, fear, and resentment would
finally take their toll. And I didn't see any effects of
depression. All I knew was I wanted to move on and
head in a new direction. I was done with the childhood
abuse and turbulent teen years. It was time for
freedom.

At eighteen, I saw nothing but promise and
possibilities. Ready to experience more, I was
determined to find what was missing. I had a plan, or
at least some idea of how I thought my life would turn
out and the person I would become. I craved success
and an exciting career, one that would make me feel
accomplished and talented. Somehow success
represented a notch on the belt of life that told the
world I had worth.

Along with my successful job, I would travel the
world. I didn't want to grow old gracefully. No way. Not
me. I had plans. It was unacceptable, even
unthinkable to live an ordinary life. I saw a great big
world out there, and I wanted to embrace it all, or at
least a large part of it. I wanted to skydive, climb
mountains, and take every form of transportation
known to mankind. I wanted to be the type of woman

o rode a motorcycle at the age of fifty, and had lots f zany adventure stories to tell her grandchildren.

This, of course, leads to the most important aspiration—a family of my own. I wanted to find a husband—the man of my dreams—a man who would make me feel whole, because it seemed like half of me was missing. I wanted that special person who would make me feel cherished and loved. Of course, I wanted children too. In my mind, giving birth to children would be my greatest achievement. When in reality it gave me stretch-marks and sleepless nights. Don't get me wrong, I'm glad I had my children. I love them dearly, but I put a tremendous burden on them the day I thought they would somehow complete me as a person.

Plans, dreams, goals, and having a vision for life are good, even vital. They can make us feel alive. The problem started, however, when I allowed those ambitions to define me. Somehow I thought career success, possessions, the right husband, and children would make me a better and complete person. Being emotionally and spiritually whole was surely found in success, marriage, and children. Finding fulfillment was wrapped inside the quest I was about to take. With high expectations, I believed without a doubt my journey would lead to everything my soul craved.

Chapter 2

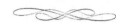

Searching in All the Wrong Places
Empty Dreams—Empty Promises

The journey I dreamed of at eighteen started to become a reality in my early twenties when I left a successful job at a thriving bank to become a travel agent. My parents were surprised at my decision, but it gave me a great opportunity to travel. I took my first cruise when I was twenty-three, and from then on, I was a world class traveler in search of adventure. Over the next five years, I took every plane, train, boat, ship and car ride I could, convinced this kind of exploration was living.

A big part of me was restless, discontent with life and who I was as a person. Looking back, I realize now I was still trying to escape the past—maybe even trying to escape from myself. Yet I must admit, when I was in some exotic place, I felt like another person— someone living out her dreams and fulfilling her expectations. I took four cruises and traveled to Hawaii, Europe, Mexico, the Caribbean, and several places across the United States. I had opportunities to travel to the South Pacific, Hong Kong, Australia, and South America. I loved it—while I was there. The trouble was, once the exciting escapade was over, I felt a deep sense of disappointment on my return. Back home, dissatisfaction set in—a letdown that caused me to hunt for the next opportunity to travel.

Desperate for the next "adventure high," I quickly planned my next trip. Travel became a drug; I couldn't get enough.

By my fifth year of travel exploration, I began to realize this lifestyle wasn't doing for me what I thought it would. I grew tired of airports and living out of a suitcase; yet, like an addict, I still wanted more. Something was missing. A void was growing in my soul and I didn't know how to fill it. Not a single exotic trip or exciting adventure ever gave me what I longed for. But I was young and I still had time to fill the longings of my soul.

Searching for Love

What is it about love, or the idea of being in love, that turns the head and heart of every girl? It's amusing, or maybe it isn't, the way many of us set ourselves up to think we need a man to be fulfilled. From early childhood, we start to believe our single most important role in life is to be a wife and mother. When we don't accomplish that goal, we feel marked as rejected, undesirable, and unacceptable.

As a teenager I remember thinking about boys, while having an idea of the type of man I wanted to marry. Funny how, as young ladies, we can develop an image of what we think "Mr. Right" will look and act like. For me, Mr. Right had to have a sense of humor. I loved to laugh, and I wanted a guy who could make me laugh even when I felt down. I didn't want a goofy clown. I wanted a sincere, tenderhearted comedian who would help me see the lighter side of life. I needed someone who was down-to-earth and easygoing, because I wasn't.

I was a hard-working perfectionist who got the job done—a Type-A personality who felt if the job had to be done right, I had to do it myself. I needed the opposite of me in order to balance my overzealous ways. I needed someone who was generous, kind, considerate, and loving—a true gentleman. I didn't expect him to be perfect, just perfect for me. As the years went by my idea of Mr. Right diminished, and I began to wonder if such a man existed.

As a teenager, finding a male companion was important. I started the search early, always yearning for that special connection. Unfortunately, while all the girls my age were dating, finding fun and new romance, I descended into deeper feelings of loneliness and rejection. I assumed if I didn't find a guy soon I was lost, doomed to wander the earth a hopeless romantic.

By the ripe old age of sixteen, I hadn't found anyone special, so I adopted the mindset that I was incomplete. Without a guy, part of me—the better half—was somehow missing, and I didn't have the foggiest idea how to replace the emptiness.

At twenty, and with the high school rejection years behind me, I suddenly had men lining up at the door. What happened? What was different? How did I go from total loser to Miss America? The truth of the matter was, I was the same person I was at fourteen, sixteen, and eighteen, I had just developed a prettier face. My once overly skinny body took on some shape, my buckteeth had been fixed with braces, and the acne finally cleared up.

Now the race was on, and I needed to make up for lost time. I had missed out on a lot of what other girls had already found, so I needed to catch up—fast. From age twenty to twenty-eight, I dated many men, some short-term, some long-term. Some I liked, others I didn't. I found dating to be fun and adventurous, yet annoying and frustrating at the same time. One of the biggest problems was the connection with each of these men, or the lack thereof. If I liked him, he didn't like me; or if he liked me, I didn't like him. This became an unrelenting cycle that often met with disappointment and aggravation.

Sometimes I dated more than one man at a time. None of those relationships were serious, but I felt this approach was necessary since I had a late start. During my all-out man hunt, I didn't sleep around. I held onto a strong sense of virtue, and I wanted to keep it. Having sex was not a price I wanted to pay to find that special man. Deep, intimate love was something I didn't want to give away to just anyone. I wanted to give myself to the one man I loved enough to walk to the altar with. Then, and only then, would it be something special.

Two men in particular engraved themselves on my heart. Some relationships not only stick with us, they change us. The trouble was, although I loved both of these men (at different times); neither of them loved me back. I poured everything I had into these relationships, yet neither offered anything of value in return. At times it made me feel as if something was wrong with me, or I wasn't good enough. I should have moved on, but their rejection made me try harder because I didn't want to let either of them go. I wanted them to see what they were giving up, that I was the best thing that could happen to them. No matter what,

I was determined to make it work. But the harder I tried, the further they ran. Both of these men knew how I felt about them, yet despite my open heart, they chose to take their love elsewhere. It took a long time to get over each of them.

Over the course of eight years, there were many ups and downs. The high points were fun, even exhilarating. The low points felt life-shattering. Yet in spite of all the good and bad, I still longed to be married and take my place in society as a woman of honor, joined to my one true love. Instead I came up empty. With my weary soul still longing, I continued to face the world alone.

Searching for Fulfillment

Life changed when I met a gentle-spirited man who was deeply in love with me. The day he offered me the marriage opportunity I was looking for, I took it. He made me feel valued and special. Like a warm blanket on a cold night, he was comfortable and inviting. His presence was a place of relaxation after a long, hard day. He was everything I longed for, or so I thought.

He wasn't the man I dreamed of, but he was tender and would do anything in his power to try and make me happy. He was intelligent, engaging, and had a way of making me laugh. Our marriage was, and still is, a good one. At this writing we've been together thirty years, and I couldn't picture myself with anyone else. Yet somehow, as good a husband and father as he is, he is not my all-in-all. Actually, no man could be.

At first, our marriage was sweet. We did well together, even though we were two very different people, and still are. He is an introvert; I am an extrovert. He is a thinker, focusing on the intellectual stimulus of the circumstance and continually looking for ways to fix things, while I allow my emotions to run on high. Frankly, I pour way too much passion into whatever situation I'm in.

When I started dating my husband, I gave up a large part of who I was as a person. I tried hard to love the things he loved, so I put the things I liked on the shelf. I loved to dance—he was uncoordinated. I loved roller coasters and adventure—he liked to stay home and watch TV. (To this day I still haven't gotten him on a roller coaster.) I liked romance and love stories—he made fun of them. He enjoyed golf—I had never held a golf club. He liked chess—I didn't understand the game. His idea of a good time was ordering pizza and watching a movie, while I was more apt to enjoy the nightlife. Somehow, through all of our differences, we made it work. I took up golf. I learned to play chess. And the nightlife went to sleep, all in exchange for what I thought would be something I truly wanted.

At first I enjoyed these new interests, and I enjoyed letting him teach me. But it didn't take long for me to wonder where my identity had gone. My name, my life, my interests and desires had suddenly become his name, his life, his interests and desires. I had somehow vanished. Instead of finding myself fulfilled in a meaningful, committed relationship, I got lost. Even though I felt we had a good marriage, my husband wasn't able to complete me the way I thought he should.

Searching for Happiness

Since neither a life of adventure nor marriage gave me what I longed for, I tried fulfilling myself with a new adventure—children. Motherhood. Could anything be better? Surely children would fill the void in my heart and give me the sense of happiness I was desperate to find. I knew from an early age I would one day be a mother. In fact, I wanted six children. I believed rearing children would be fun, a virtual playground of exciting moments filled with laughter and good times. I had no idea what I was getting myself into.

My husband and I talked about having children before we got married. So for us it was a natural course of action. However, since I was closing in on the age of thirty, I worried there wouldn't be enough time to bear all the children we wanted. I felt we needed to get started right away. My biological clock was ticking and soon became a loud drum in my hungry soul.

We weren't married a year when I became pregnant for the first time. Looking back, this became one of my biggest regrets—having children too soon after our marriage began. I don't see the pregnancy as a mistake. I just wish we had more time to be a couple before we dove into the extended family plan. Over the next ten years, I became pregnant three more times, and we were blessed with three beautiful, healthy children: two girls and a boy. Our fourth child died while still in the womb.

The miscarriage was very difficult. I was well into the pregnancy, so when I lost the baby, people noticed. Somehow kind and encouraging people didn't know how to act around me. I can't say I blame them. What do you say when one of the mothers at your daughter's ballet class is obviously pregnant, and the next week she isn't?

The first couple of days afterward, it felt as though I were walking through a thick, blinding fog. Suddenly, I was an actor playing a part on stage and nothing around me was real. To some degree, this feeling of detachment helped me cope. By the third day, hormones took over, and I began to have crying spells. A tidal wave of thoughts and emotions overtook my soul as I began to grasp the depth of our loss. Through the heart-wrenching days that followed, I didn't think I would pull through. Then one day I received a phone call from the hospital informing me of the autopsy results. Apparently, our daughter's spinal cord wasn't attached to her brain, so even if she had lived, she would have been completely unable to do anything. This news was devastating, yet in time my soul was freed to find peace. To this day I can still feel the loss, but there came a point when I was able to release her, able to accept the hope she was in a better place.

. Many years have come and gone since that time, and as a family, we've been through a great deal. My children are grown now and having children of their own. For the most part, I enjoyed my children and still do. But like everything else in life, my children did not fill the emptiness in my heart. I had unknowingly placed an unfair burden on them by assigning them an impossible task. They could never shape me into the person I was meant to be.

So if travel adventures, marriage, and motherhood weren't going to make me happy and fill the longings of my soul, then what would? If these things couldn't give me meaning and purpose in life, then where could I find it?

Searching for Success

In the world's eyes, carrying the banner of a successful career brings prestige, honor, and recognition that cannot be found anywhere else. Such success includes titles, accolades, rewards, and lots of money. A high-ranking, successful career can be a launching pad to many great things in life, and denotes those who accomplish it as a man or woman of greatness. When people look at someone who is successful, they are filled with awe and respect; perceiving this person as one of exceptional importance. Who wouldn't want the privilege of being held in high esteem?

What pressure I put on myself, and allowed the world to put on me, when I craved this kind of prestige. In those days, I thought reaching and striving for success would make me happy, satisfied, and content. It would somehow place me in a well-deserved category that would give me a level of accomplishment everyone would not only appreciate but value. I wanted to be somebody, to make my mark on the world. I wanted to find a sense of purpose. Basically, I wanted to matter.

Before my so-called "successful" career days, when my days were filled with the daily responsibilities of marriage and motherhood, I would encounter career women who would inevitably ask me the question: "So, what do you do?" I always dreaded this question, because every time I gave the normal response of, "I'm a wife and mother," I felt looked down upon. Even though I had worked in the business world for ten years prior to marriage, and was pursuing higher education, marriage and children abruptly, and without warning, sent me from someone of value to someone insignificant. Within seconds of my "housewife" declaration, I found myself an outsider, an outcast among the professional women in the room.

When this happened I became disappointed, even disillusioned, about my role as a young mother. Suddenly, I didn't measure up, and felt less of a woman. At that time, I didn't have a clear understanding or value of my purpose in the extraordinary role of motherhood. So as the days and months went by, I became disheartened and bored; I even convinced myself what I was doing wasn't worthwhile.

A growing sadness developed within me that made me feel lost in the mundane routine of wiping noses, watching Barney for the millionth time, and preparing yet another peanut butter and jelly sandwich. Somewhere between changing diapers and endless loads of laundry, I lost the sense of who I was again, and began to wonder what happened to that energetic young woman, who at one time was full of hopes and dreams.

Now that I am an older mother, long past the disappointment and disillusionment that told me my children should somehow complete me, I now see clearly. Yes, my children are a mark on this world, they are a part of me, and I am a reflection of them, but they are not my all-in-all. Since then I have come to realize being a mother is the hardest and most demanding job I could ever have. Looking back, I am amazed, even a little ashamed, to have allowed those other women to determine my worth based on a corporate job description. Being a mother is the most important job I've ever had. No other career, job, or project I've taken on has equaled it, or can compare to its high level of dedication and commitment. I'm only sorry it took me so long to learn that lesson.

From the time I entered the working world, I worked many jobs, and for the most part did well at everything I put my hands on. I earned that college degree, with honors, all while renovating a hundred-year-old Victorian with my husband and giving birth to our two daughters. I was seven months pregnant with our son the day I received my diploma. Our graduation gowns were silver, and I looked like a torpedo walking down the aisle.

In the working world, both before and after marriage, I won awards, was given promotions, and placed in positions of leadership. I was recognized before multitudes, and my company named me their number one sales consultant in the area I served. I earned a car, received admiration from my colleagues, and was accepted with open arms into many well-respected organizations. In the world's eyes, I was successful.

Unfortunately, the more success I found, the more miserable I became. It didn't make sense. This wasn't how it was supposed to be. Where was that sense of accomplishment and purpose? Why was I still feeling empty, frustrated, and discouraged? Why couldn't I find myself and my reason for living?

Chapter 3

Where Did I Go Wrong?
Hiding the Hurt, Masking the Pain

By the time I turned thirty-five, I had everything: a husband who loved me, three beautiful, healthy children, a nice house, and a successful career. I was experiencing success in every area of life, and I worked hard to convince myself I was happy. My schedule was full of activities, programs, and projects. Externally I had it all, but inwardly I was discontent.

Wasn't all of this success supposed to make me feel good? Wasn't all my achievement and activity supposed to validate me as a person of worth? Why did I feel dissatisfied? A man, children, money, career—none of it brought me the happiness and fulfillment I craved. Part of my problem was false expectation. Even though I had everything I longed for and set out to achieve from the time I was eighteen, once I received it, it didn't measure up—it couldn't. I tried to lay hold of every hope, dream, and expectation this world taught me to pursue, only to come up empty.

For all this time I allowed a world that didn't have the faintest idea how to live tell me how to live. I believed the lie. I was sold on the idea of what a perfect life is supposed to look like. So when I reached what should have been a high point in life, when everything should have been perfect, instead of celebrating, I fell apart.

When I assumed the world's way of doing things would define me as the person I was meant to be, I set the stage for ultimate unhappiness. I put all my hopes and dreams into what I thought would deliver great reward, only to find the rug pulled out from under me—leaving me crushed in a crescendo of disappointments, dashed dreams, and misguided expectations.

What should have been my greatest journey toward satisfaction turned out to be my worst nightmare. Nothing made me happy. Nothing made me whole. Nothing gave me the sense of life, love, and purpose I frantically sought after. For seventeen years I searched for life, love, and happiness in all the wrong places. In an attempt to find myself—I lost myself. I didn't have a clue where to turn.

Believing the Lies

Even though I was falling apart emotionally and spiritually, I didn't want to admit it. Admitting my inner (wo)man was a mess meant failure. Outwardly I had it all, so how could I tell others I was miserable? It was not okay for me to exhibit a great life and then say, "I'm not okay;" at least not out loud. So I lied. Every day I wore a thin mask of confidence.

I was nothing more than an archetype for the walking wounded, wearing a smile while secretly screaming, "Help!" I was an actor, a true veteran of the stage, and Hollywood had nothing on me. My performance was so flawless no one could tell what was really going on—not even me.

My friends frequently commented on how well I held everything together and seemed at ease while doing it. They couldn't see the ticking time bomb ready to explode. But there came a day when I could no longer put on the mask and play the role I thought I was assigned. Without warning, a foreigner took my place on stage, someone I didn't know—someone I had never met before—and she acted nothing like me.

Hiding the Pain

Sometimes we can be fooled by the way a person carries herself in public, by the way she speaks, dresses, or acts, and come to the conclusion she has no problems. This is always a lie. All people have problems. Some are just better at wearing the mask. The thought that anyone has it all together now scares me. In fact, I've learned that those who most look as if they have it all together may be the very ones who don't. Millions of people live with depression, yet you wouldn't know it because they hide the pain well. Depression comes with a stigma; a label no one wants to carry. Regrettably for some, the truth is revealed after it's too late.

A friend of mine worked with a middle-aged man, who on the surface appeared to have it all. He was wealthy, well-educated and well-dressed. He had a lovely wife and two grown children. He lived in an upscale neighborhood and was the CEO of a company. Yet no one he worked with knew he battled depression. Until one day, a perfectly normal day, filled with meetings, phone calls, and a solid return on the company's investments, this man went home and shot himself. Everyone was stunned, completely unable to comprehend the idea that this man was anything but happy.

Another man I know shared his story with me. "It was the worst year of my life," he began. In 2008, when the economy came crashing down, many people lost everything. Some lost their jobs, their homes, their financial security, and their hopes for the future. This man was no different. In order to survive, he sold everything he could. His business was in trouble, but he refused to give up and desperately tried to hold onto a few remaining employees.

"I pretended everything was okay," he continued. "I had everyone fooled. No one knew how bad the company's finances were. I lost almost everything, but I did everything I could to hold onto my business." Before the year was out, he hit rock bottom—flat broke, in deep financial debt, and the company didn't earn a penny that year. He became so depressed he lost the will to live. Thankfully, he survived, but not one person in his life knew the heavy burden he carried.

Odds are each of us knows someone suffering with depression, but sometimes we aren't aware of it. We work with them, maybe even live with them, yet we miss it, completely unable to recognize the signs. Depression does give off many clues, but unless we're familiar with depression, it can go undetected until something drastic happens.

Just because I looked as if I had it all together didn't mean I did. People bought into the lie that *Patty was above reproach, heartache, and the basic troubles of life.* I was afraid that if people really knew me and saw who I was underneath, they wouldn't like me anymore. So for a long time I suffered in silence.

One of the biggest reasons I didn't open up at first about how I was feeling was because I didn't trust anyone. And I wasn't ready to become vulnerable. Vulnerability made me feel weak and frightened, so I would not lay my soul bare before others. Deep inside though, part of me longed for someone to listen, to understand and offer help and encouragement, to tell me everything would be okay. Yet day-after-day, I continued to hide.

Chapter 4

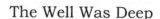

The Well Was Deep

Struggling to Find a Way Out

Then came the day I began to realize I was depressed. Standing onstage in Dallas, Texas, before thousands, being recognized for one of the highest levels of achievement in the company, I found myself thinking: *Is this all there is?* Abruptly, everything I poured myself into that year didn't make sense. As I stood on that stage, listening to the loud music and thunderous applause, I began to think: *Is this what I shipped my children off to a babysitter for? Is this why I did the changing of the guard with my husband?* (When he came home from work, I went off to work. I hardly saw him that year.)

In the middle of what should have been a magnificent moment, my soul began its plummet from this momentary high, to miserable depths of confusion.

On the flight home, hot tears of frustration and anger welled in my eyes. At the peak of success, the height of what should have been my finest hour, I hit a wall and began spiraling down a deep, dark tunnel. Suddenly nothing I had accomplished mattered anymore.

In the days that followed the conference, I began to turn my back on everything and everyone I thought would bring me happiness. I found fault and became critical of everything my husband and children did, or didn't do. Nothing was good enough; and no matter how hard my family tried to please me, they couldn't gain my approval. And the career I once loved became a huge, pointless waste of time.

I wandered through each day like a blind beggar, not knowing what I was begging for. Nothing helped. No matter what I did in an attempt to feel better, it didn't work. I couldn't get past the overwhelming feelings of sadness and worthlessness. Each day grew increasingly harder, every minute increasingly darker. I felt helpless, like a prisoner trapped in my own body.

As the emotional turmoil of depression grew, patterns of rage reemerged. In my teen years, bits and pieces of repressed emotions surfaced, but they were nothing compared to what came out now. As those suppressed feelings escalated to their full potential, it was frightening—even to me. I had never felt anything like this before. The outbursts of anger made me feel ugly, as if something dark and evil had overtaken my body. At times I was so enraged, I was ready to put my fist through a wall. Fortunately, I didn't. But that was the level of wrath venting in my heart and mind. Looking back, I justified those bouts of fury, convinced they gave me some kind of control over a situation that was completely out of control. The truth was, I was frightened and had no idea how to control or reverse what was ruining my life. I was confused by the emotional pain and didn't understand where it was coming from.

As the depression intensified, so did my bouts of rage. The one who was hit the hardest was my oldest daughter. Often without warning I attacked her verbally and physically. The brunt of the abuse

happened while she was very young. I don't know wh
I focused my fury on her. I didn't lash out at my other
two children. Maybe because, like me, she was the
oldest. Maybe I saw a reflection of myself in her, a
defenseless child on whom I could take out my hurt
and anger. Perhaps I was lashing out because I saw
her as a substitute for my problems. Maybe I was
acting out in revenge, doing to her what I wanted to do
to those who had hurt me.

I never sought therapy for what I had gone
through as a child. I never asked for professional
advice about any of the repressed feelings I harbored. I
was oblivious and thought I was over the past hurts
and had moved on in my search of a better life. But as
the life I dreamed of let me down, the old feelings and
hurts came back, flooding my soul with pain. I felt
terrified of who I had become. I didn't know who to
turn to or what to do. So when I became abusive to my
daughter, I was too afraid to tell anyone. I needed
help, but any time I thought about getting help, my
first thought was, *They'll take her away.*

As the days dragged into months, I helplessly sank
deeper and deeper into a well of depression. I spent
my days sleeping, screaming, and crying, as a sense of
defeat and frustration grew within my soul.

In the midst of all this anguish, alcohol became
my solitary source of comfort. It wasn't much at first,
a drink or two at night after I put the children to bed.
Sitting beside my husband watching TV, sipping a
small glass of wine numbed me and made me feel
calmer. It was a lie, but I convinced myself the alcohol
had temporarily relieved the darkness.

ιe alcohol made a difference in the way I
ιed, I started to drink earlier and more
... ι reached a point where I didn't want to feel
anything anymore—not angry or depressed—and the
alcohol helped me deal with both. By mid-afternoon
each day, I began pouring that first glass of numbing
therapy, and continued to drink until late in the
evening to help divert the turmoil. The alcohol also
made me sleepy, providing another form of escape.

A Portrait of Depression

To sidestep a little, I want to give you another
picture of depression. If you're familiar with the Bible,
you may know about a story found in Jeremiah[3],
where several men threw Jeremiah into a cistern and
left him there alone to starve to death. The well was
deep, and mud filled the bottom, which made it
impossible for Jeremiah to free himself. With every
attempt to climb out, he only sank deeper into the
mud.

Depression is like being thrown into that cistern,
where there is nothing except darkness, dirt, and
mud. You can see yourself struggling to get out,
fighting hard to climb the dirt walls, clawing and
digging, only to have pieces of dirt come lose and fall
into your eyes and mouth. You lift one leg to try and
find a foothold, only to have the other leg plunge
deeper into the suctioning mud. You hear yourself
calling out, screaming for help. In the gloom, you hear
nothing except the sound of your own voice as it
echoes in the murky pit. Again and again you call out,
but no one hears. No one comes. It doesn't take long
before you come to the conclusion that every effort is

futile. There is no answer and no hope of getting out, so you sit down in the mud, surrounded by the gloomy shadows of your hollow tomb, and wait to die.

If you know what it is to struggle with depression, you can relate to Jeremiah all too well.

I knew how I felt when I was in that well, and I wondered if Jeremiah felt the same things I did? He must have. When he was thrown into the well, he must have been confused as to why the men put him there. He surely reasoned with them in an attempt to stop their cruelty. He must have called out, hoping someone might be passing by and hear him. I'll bet he called out several times, maybe even day-after-day, night-after-night for deliverance. He must have held onto the hope that one of his friends or family members would realize he was missing and search for him. And maybe felt betrayed when the people in his life didn't come to his aid. Jeremiah undoubtedly searched for a way out. But I wonder, as he struggled to free himself, when all his efforts failed, did he too come to the conclusion his situation was hopeless?

When I was in the well, I made every effort I could think of to find answers—to get better—to stop feeling the way I did, but with each attempt, failure was the only outcome. It was difficult to come to the conclusion I couldn't free myself from the emotional turmoil. I had to look beyond myself to find relief. I had to open my heart and tell people something was wrong, and I needed help. As a private person, I rarely spoke of personal matters with anyone, but with the depression deepening, I couldn't wait any longer. I had to take the risk.

No One Understood

I was afraid of what others would think. How would they react when I told them about my extreme sadness, bouts of rage, the abuse, and turning to alcohol to cope? Would they judge me, criticize my feelings and condemn my actions? Would they stop loving me, or stop being my friend?

Until this point, no one, not even my husband, knew about the pain, my abuse toward our oldest daughter, or the excessive drinking—I hid it all too well. So when I finally found the courage to start talking about what I was going through, to my surprise, no one judged, criticized, or condemned. Instead they didn't believe me. I was confused why no one took me seriously. I couldn't figure out why no one seemed to understand or even listen.

I felt betrayed by the people I loved. Ironically, those whom I previously helped and supported didn't seem concerned. It broke my heart to think how I had been there when life knocked them down. I was the bailout queen, the one everyone turned to for help in picking up the pieces of their shattered lives. Countless times I listened, gave money, lent a hand, or offered assistance. It was not a burden, I wanted to help. It was the nature of my heart, and I never expected anything in return. But the hurt was beyond words when I was in trouble and needed help, and *no one* came to my aid.

During the depression I never felt lonelier. Feeling cheated, I told myself that people only wanted to be around me if I had something to give. I didn't want to be around anyone who told me they loved me one minute, then turned their back on me the next. The love in my heart quickly grew cold.

Even my sweet husband didn't get it. Night after night I tried to tell him something was wrong. And every time he said, "Oh, you'll get over it." I knew my husband loved me, but he hadn't gone through depression himself. He couldn't identify with the pain, so he didn't understand what I was going through.

My husband telling me to "get over it" never helped me "get over it." I don't know why he made that assumption, but he was the type of guy who wanted to fix everything, and perhaps this was his way of fixing my problems. But no matter how hard I tried, I couldn't "get over it." Believe me, if I could have controlled those overwhelming feelings of anger, sadness and despair, I would have. What I needed from my husband was compassion. I needed an active listener with whom I could be open and transparent, someone to really hear what I was going through and try to comfort me. But his lack of understanding only made me feel worse, and hopeless.

Nowhere to Turn

Hopeless—is there any word in the English language more dreadful? After I exhausted all efforts to find help through family and friends, I turned to the medical profession for relief. At first, whenever I brought up the subject, my husband was against it. He was convinced I was fine and didn't want me to seek professional help. He thought my seeing a doctor would somehow disparage his career, or put him in a position to be compromised for having a crazy wife. But his lack of empathy and understanding was not going to stop me. So I took every opportunity to set a little money aside so when I accumulated enough to pay cash, I'd call and make an appointment under an assumed name. No one would ever know.

A few months later I picked up the phone in order to follow through with my well-laid plan. With phonebook in hand, and a get-fixed-quick mentality, I called one doctor's office after another, bent on the mission that if I could get some pills, I'd be fine. But the responses I got were all like: "I'm sorry, we don't take your insurance." Or, "I'm sorry, we don't handle that kind of depression."

In less than an hour, I had made my way through the entire list of professional doctors I thought could help me. Finally, when I dialed the last number on the list, a kind woman answered the phone and listened patiently to my heartfelt plea, only to tell me, at the end of our conversation, "I'm sorry, but we can't help you." As I hung up the phone a thought swiftly dawned on me: *No one can help me—I'm utterly alone. This is never going to end.* At that moment the darkness went deeper, and thoughts of suicide invaded my mind.

Chapter 5

<hr/>

God Had Other Plans

Turning Something Bad into Something Good

Hopelessness turned into utter desperation when I realized no one could help me. I had no friends, family, or medical support to turn to, so that opened the way for thoughts of suicide to fill my mind. The mind is vulnerable, and when in a state of hopelessness can come up with endless scenarios that are neither right nor healthy. But at this point, I no longer cared. I just wanted the madness to end, so I gave up, quit trying, and began to tell myself the only way out was to die.

In the days that followed, I found myself doing something I rarely did—I prayed. Praying to a God I didn't know felt foreign, but I didn't know what else to do. I was desperate to end the pain, but I didn't pray for God's help, mercy, or healing. Nor did I call on him to find answers. I asked him to take my life. He had the power to make me live or die—and I wanted to die. Every morning I prayed for the insanity to end, and every night I prayed to never wake up. In the afternoons I would lie down with the same prayer on my mind, *Please, God, just let me die.*

One sunny day in November, after picking up the kids from the babysitter, I put a video in for my young daughters and took my toddler son upstairs and put him in his crib. Once the kids were set, I went into my bedroom, lay down on the bed, fully dressed, ready to die. I couldn't take it anymore. My life felt like hell on earth—an endless misery of destruction I couldn't escape. As I closed my eyes, my heart again pleaded with God to take my life. Instead, within seconds, I fell asleep.

An hour later I woke up to face the disappointment that God had not answered my prayer. Frustrated and angry, I got up grumbling at him. *Why are you not letting me die? Surely this is not an impossible task. Can't you see how useless my life has become?*

Then I looked in on my son, still asleep in his crib. Downstairs, the girls were exactly where I had left them, sitting quietly in front of the television, watching a movie. At the time I didn't think about the consequences of leaving three young children unattended. Now I recognize the grace and mercy that had been at work while I slept off the effects of another emotional breakdown. I believe God sent angels to watch over my children. Yet in the middle of my ranting and ungrateful heart, I neither recognized nor appreciated the gift he had given me.

Depression is blinding, like trying to move through a dark room in the middle of the night. It was like the time I was six years old, playing blind-man's-bluff with my seven cousins on my uncle's back porch. It was nighttime, and since we didn't turn a light on, it was very dark—and of course I was the one wearing the blindfold. Being kids, none of us had checked for hazards prior to playing the game, and we didn't realize the cellar door had been left open. Cellar doors, unlike basement doors, are in the floor not the wall. As the game progressed, I called out as my cousins taunted me toward their direction. I moved cautiously around the porch, but not cautious enough. Without warning, I stepped into the opening of the cellar and plummeted to the concrete floor below—and I blacked out. I woke up in Dad's arms as he carried me up the cellar stairs. Thankfully, I didn't suffer any permanent damage as a result of the fall, but I could have died.

With no light to guide me through the darkness of depression, I couldn't see what was right in front of me. I didn't have the capability to recognize anything good in my life. Many wonderful things happened, but I couldn't see any of them, probably because I didn't want to. Nor could I see the dangers of the lifestyle I had chosen to cope with the pain.

I lost a great deal because of the depression. One of my biggest regrets was the time I lost with my children. I cared for them but only did what was needed. My children became hostages in their own home. Other than school, I don't remember taking them anywhere or doing anything with them. I didn't play with them. I only popped in one video after another to keep the girls occupied, and kept my son in his crib. I have very little record of their childhood during that time. I took all kinds of pictures and videos of the girls when they were babies. But there were very few baby photos of my son or the girls during this time. I was too emotionally ill to pick up a camera. I regret the time and memories that we lost, but at the time it didn't matter—nothing mattered.

Nothing Left to Give

Convinced everyone would be better off without me, I planned to take my life. Although my children were six, four, and one, I actually believed I would be doing them a favor. With me in the picture, their lives were in constant upheaval. With all my screaming, crying, and fits of rage, life for them was dreadful. I knew committing suicide was wrong and that my actions would hurt my family tremendously, but the darkness was so thick and heavy, I didn't see another answer. Death seemed to be the only way any of us would find peace.

I rehearsed several different scenarios, trying to think of the best way to accomplish the goal. Being a strategic, well-organized woman, I treated the plan as I would any other situation. There was a lot to consider, and I wanted to make this as easy on my family as possible.

The most crucial point came on December 12, 1996. I couldn't go on one more day. Waking up that morning, I felt my heart harden even more toward God for forcing me to face another day. As I lay in bed, staring at the ceiling, I thought, *Why won't you let me die?*

Reluctantly, I got up and stepped into the shower, my hot tears mixed with the hot water. Naked, drenched, and ashamed, I felt I had been ground into the ashes from which I came. Nothing was left of me. I had reached my end. Yet through the sobs, I began to talk to God. "I have nowhere else to go but you. You have to do something. No one can help me; only you can help me. Please, help me!"

This was a total change from my previous cries. This time I asked for a miracle. As I cried out I knew this was a desperate make-it-or-break-it moment. If God didn't do something that day, I feared I would. My plea was not an ultimatum. I wasn't bargaining with

God. I had hit rock bottom. I was desperate with nowhere else to go.

Suddenly, through the sobs, my ears heard what sounded like a faint voice, "Go to MOPS." (MOPS stands for Mothers of Preschoolers, a Christian women's organization that ministers to women who have children ages five and under.) At first I moaned because I wasn't in any mood to be around people. I already belonged to the organization, so I was already assigned to sit with a group of women. But because of the depression, I had been avoiding the meetings. As my emotions tried to persuade me to stay home, I heard the voice again, "Go to MOPS."

So I got out of the shower, got dressed, dropped the girls off at school, and went to MOPS with my son. Once there, I put on the mask that told the other moms I was fine. I was struggling to keep myself together, but the last thing I wanted to do was let the ladies at the church think I wasn't doing well. I didn't want them to know about the rage and emotional turmoil, and I certainly didn't want them to know about the depression or my suicidal tendencies.

As the meeting began, I was like an elegant dancer who had practiced her part so well, she performed it with perfect execution. I smiled, even laughed a few times. I ate, conversed with the other moms, and even put together a craft. Which, by the way, I hate to do.

Toward the latter part of our MOPS gathering, the speaker came forward and stood behind the podium. She was an older woman, maybe in her mid-sixties. She was plain, yet lovely with a quiet, gentle spirit. When she began to speak, her demeanor was light and entertaining. Her mix of humor and grace caught my attention, and I found myself enjoying her tremendously. She shared some things about her life, and even talked about her husband who had Parkinson's disease. But she commanded my full attention when she shared about what it's like to have a lack of joy and no real purpose in life. She didn't specifically talk about depression, but what she said fell in line with how I was feeling. The real crux of her message was about finding joy and purpose in life and that the only way to find pure joy was through Jesus Christ. I was intrigued and found myself hanging on her every word. As she closed, she told the group about a brochure she had, and if anyone wanted one, to meet her afterward.

As she made her way to the back of the room, I got up and quickly followed her, convinced I needed a brochure. She looked at me and smiled warmly. I don't remember how the conversation started or how I got to the point of hysterics, but before I knew it, and without warning, an emotional dam broke, and I found myself rambling and sobbing uncontrollably in front of her, trying desperately to form coherent sentences.

She didn't say a word as I rambled through the frantic outburst. I couldn't control what was happening. I couldn't stop crying, couldn't stop talking, not even when I realized every woman in the room had turned around to stare at us. But I didn't care. At that moment, I no longer cared who knew or what anyone thought. It didn't matter anymore. I needed help, and this woman in front of me had the answer. I was tired of holding all the pain inside. I wanted it out and didn't care how. I just wanted the emotional madness to end.

In the midst of my ranting, she seemed to care, even though she had never met me before. Somehow I sensed she understood the pain, knew what I was dealing with and wanted to help.

Quietly she listened for several minutes. Then without saying a word, she touched me on my left arm and when she did the hysterics, crying, and run-on sentences instantly stopped—as if someone had shut off a running faucet. With just one touch of her hand there was no more nausea in the pit of my stomach. The dark cloud that had been my constant companion was gone. The heaviness lifted—everything—all of the darkness that had consumed my life was completely gone. My spirit and soul felt light, as if they had taken on wings and could fly around the room. For the first time in my life, I felt freedom. I didn't understand what had happened. I was stunned, completely amazed. I stood there and stared at her, frozen by what had just taken place.

I had no idea if she knew what had happened, because she still didn't say a word. Yet there was something about her I had never known before, and as I looked into her eyes, I could see great love and tender compassion. Silently, I turned and walked away, my mind filling with thoughts as I desperately tried to comprehend the experience. I knew this woman did not possess the power to heal me, but I believed God did. Even though I didn't understand what had happened, I was convinced the power I felt rush through me had to be God.

Finding Freedom

That morning in the shower, when I cried out to God, I believe he heard me and orchestrated this deliverance. There was no other explanation. He healed me, just as he had healed so many others in biblical times, and still does today. His touch through this woman lifted the darkness. My brokenness invited him, and by acknowledging my need for him, it qualified me for his touch. I had nothing left to give but brokenness, yet that was what he had been waiting for. When I tore off the mask and became honest with God, he heard my cry. He wanted to set me free from the suffering; he just had another way of ending it. I thought the only way out was death, but God had other plans. When I saw only devastation in my life, God saw promise. When I saw only hopelessness, God saw a way to bring me near. To me the depression felt like the end. To God the depression was the beginning of a whole new life with him.

Chapter 6

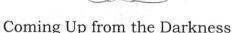

Coming Up from the Darkness

Release from the Pain

The week that followed I felt nothing but joy. My world went from deep depression, emptiness, and devastation, to utter exuberance. Instantly, my life rose from the ashes and burst with delight. I had found hope. Laughter and joy filled my heart, and a sense of pleasure overtook my soul.

When Jesus reached into my depraved world, he turned everything right side up. The transformation was undeniable. Everyone close to me noticed. One night in particular, standing at the stove cooking dinner, I heard my husband call from the other room, "What's that sound?" That sound was my singing! The joy in my voice was something he had never heard before.

At last, things were changing in the Mason home. Laughter found its way in, and what had once been a house full of fear, misery, anger and sadness became a home filled with fresh love. And everyone living within its walls could finally relax.

The Freedom Kept Coming

Although I was now beginning to live the life I had once dreamed about, God had more in mind. It wasn't enough for me to find his joy—he wanted me to find him. He wanted me to know more than the goodness of his mercy and compassion through the healing. He wanted me to know his intimate love through a personal relationship.

During that first week, I couldn't stop thinking about Jesus. This was strange since prior to the depression, I had never given God much thought. I believed in Jesus and that he died on the cross, but I didn't have any connection to him. I rarely prayed, except when I was desperate. I never read the Bible. I went to church when I felt like it, which was seldom. I called a friend who put Jesus at the center of her life a fanatic. But after the healing, my attitude changed. I became grateful for what Jesus had done. I couldn't let go of him, or the mercy he had shown me.

Then on December 18, 1996, six days after the eventful MOPS experience, Jesus brought more into my life than I had ever thought possible. It became a turning point that would leave its mark on my life forever.

At four o'clock that afternoon, as I waited for my children getting haircuts at a local salon, I noticed a poster on the wall advertising a Christmas play at a nearby church. I felt we had to go. The program was at 7 o'clock. By the time my children were finished, it was almost 5 o'clock. I quickly put them in the car and drove to the church to see if tickets were still available. Since it was late in the afternoon, only the church secretary was in the office. She smiled warmly when I walked into the room.

"Do you have any tickets left for tonight's performance?" I asked.

"No, I'm sorry," she replied. "We're all sold out."

Heartbroken, I thanked her and turned to leave. But before I crossed the threshold, she called out, "But come anyway. Come early and we'll find you a seat."

Overjoyed, I hurried home, quickly made dinner, got ready, and headed back to the church with my daughters in tow.

The church was packed. Yet even with no tickets, the usher politely guided us to three available seats in the balcony. Sitting high above the main floor, we could easily see everything.

The program was broken into four unique performances. The first was a singing Christmas tree. About thirty members of the choir, all dressed in green, stood in such a way that they formed a giant Christmas tree. This group sang the newer contemporary Christmas songs. In the second portion, the singers looked like characters who had strolled off the set of an adaption of Charles Dickens' *A Christmas Carol*. The songs they sang were more traditional and time-honored. The third segment was full of childhood wonders, reminiscent of *Babes in Toyland*.

For the final act, the church reenacted the birth of Jesus. As a child growing up in the sixties, I had seen the reenactment several times on television. Back then it was acceptable to show traditional Christmas programming on regular network stations. So I watched Christmas programs like *Nester the Long-Eared Christmas Donkey* and *The Little Drummer Boy*. Yet none of what I'd seen before touched me the way this did. It was as if I was seeing the birth of Jesus for the first time. I wept at all the sights and sounds. I felt as though I was a part of what was happening.

When the program ended, the senior pastor took the stage and began to talk about God's grace, his redemptive love, and how the only way to find salvation was through Jesus. Although I had grown up attending a traditional church, I had no idea what he was talking about. I didn't remember anyone having talked about salvation. I remembered being called a sinner, but didn't understand I was separated from God due to sin. I believed Jesus died on the cross. Yet I was unaware of the extent of God's grace, mercy, and love offered to me by faith through Jesus.

My exposure to church had been punitive. As a child I saw church as nothing more than religion based on burdensome rules and mechanical rituals, not a place to find love and acceptance. Church intimidated me and often left me feeling worse than when I had arrived. So when I became old enough to make my own decisions, I only went on holidays and rare occasions.

But now everything felt different. Because of the miraculous freedom I now tasted, my closed heart swung wide open. So when the pastor asked if anyone wanted to receive Jesus by faith as their personal Savior, I didn't hesitate to say, "Yes!" My response was not out of duty or obligation, or even a sense of gratitude. I didn't understand everything. I had no idea what all of this meant—all I knew, all I understood, was I needed Jesus. And that was enough.

With newfound courage and faith, as the pastor prayed what some call the "sinner's prayer," I echoed his every word. Heavy tears streaked my face as I opened my heart to receive Jesus into my life. I would never be the same. Just like the healing, saying "yes" to Jesus was a new beginning, a fresh start in a life that was once drowning in darkness.

Since That Day

Once Jesus became my personal Savior, he began a deeper work that changed my heart, old attitudes, and life in ways I never dreamed possible. He began to take all my striving, all my efforts to find happiness and self-worth, and offered me something of greater value. I went from looking for love in all the wrong places to knowing true love.[4] I went from wearing the mask, trying to be perfect in a flawed world, to resting in the assurance that I am fearfully and wonderfully made.[5] I went from having no hope to having a hope and a future.[6] For years, I felt part of me was missing. In order to find myself I pursued what I thought would fill me—a man, children, money, travel, and a successful career. For seventeen years I went on one quest after another in an attempt to find what my soul longed for, but each time I ended up disappointed and empty. This world had nothing to offer me, yet every time I allowed the world and its views to fill me in some way, the results were unsatisfying and left an ache in my soul.

What I didn't realize when God formed us, he created us with a God-sized void *only he* can fill. So every time I went in search of what I thought would fill me, I felt empty and incomplete, because none of those things could take God's place.

You and I can search the world trying to fill that God-sized void—joining ourselves to whatever we think will fill us: people, family, possessions, money, goals, plans, dreams, desires, success, accomplishments, power, comfort, acceptance, addiction, any number of things. But every time we do, we will come away empty and unsatisfied. We may find a temporary quick fix now and then that will give us a false sense of satisfaction, but it will not take long for the momentary thrill to wear off and send us right back to feeling unfulfilled.

All the striving and struggling to find worth and fulfillment began to shift when Jesus entered my life. As my relationship with him deepened, I started to find new meaning and a reason to live. My life now had direction and a true sense of determination that was leading me down paths I never dreamed I would take. If you told me prior to the depression that I would one day be an author and speaker involved in ministry, I probably would have laughed. Even though I didn't see myself this way, God did. He knew the plans he had for me long before I was born. He knew what he desired to accomplish in my life, and he knew the path I would have to take to find my way to those purposes. God knew from the beginning how to win my heart, draw me close to himself, and bring me into the plans he had for me.

I was once like Jeremiah, unwillingly thrown into a deep, dark well with no way out. But Jeremiah didn't die in that well, and neither did I, even though I thought I would. The Bible doesn't tell us how long Jeremiah was trapped in the well, but as we read the story we learn, at some point, Ebed-Melek, which means the "king's servant," heard what had happened and spoke to the king. So the king told Ebed-Melek to take thirty men and lift Jeremiah from the well. The men went to a room under the king's treasury and found some rags and old clothes. They tied those rags together and let them down with some rope to Jeremiah. They told him what to do, and then lifted Jeremiah from the well.[7]

Jesus himself reached into my well and pulled me out. And when he did, I came out a different person. Then, over time, he taught me how to take the things found in his rich treasury, tie them together, and let them down into the well for others who are trapped— helping them to see the power of God's truth, love, mercy and grace—so they too can find hope, healing, and freedom for their wounded and weary souls.

Does God Really Care?

Right now you may be thinking, *That's great, I'm glad God healed you, but what about me? Does God really care about me?*

Whether you know God or not, sometimes, when you've suffered for a long time, it's hard to believe that God loves you and cares about you. Sometimes when you've been through so much, it's hard to accept the truth that God has a plan and purpose for your life.

The world wasn't always the way we see it today. In the beginning, when God created the world, it was perfect. There was no pain, no disease, no death, and *no depression*. But when mankind turned away from God and turned toward his own way, sin entered the perfect world God created which in turn caused a ripple effect, bringing all kinds of suffering into the world.[8]

But God had a plan to restore what was lost—to restore the relationship he once shared with mankind in the Garden of Eden. That's why God sent Jesus, his one and only Son, to take all our sin upon himself and die for us, and then be raised to life again. By taking our sin upon himself and carrying it to the cross, Jesus made a way for us to find forgiveness, through which we can find hope and healing from our wandering. By his resurrection, we are given a new life and brought back into the relationship God longs for us to share with him.[9] For Jesus didn't come to condemn the world, but so that through him the world might be saved.[10]

You may have questions and are struggling to find answers, but no matter what you feel, there is one constant truth: *God loves you and cares about you.* Right now the darkness may be so deep and thick you can't see or feel his love. But God is with you in the darkness. He sees you. He knows your pain and every tear you cry. He watches over you and longs for the moment you will give your heart to him.

Maybe, like me, you have been searching, pursuing the things you thought would satisfy you and make you happy. Maybe you're trying to fill that void in your soul, or masking the depression with addiction. What are you looking for? What's missing? What are you turning to? No matter what it is, the answer is Jesus.

I'm not trying to preach to you. I am a simple woman who found love, acceptance, peace, joy, and healing through the heart of a Savior who was willing to save her. My purpose in sharing these things is not to convert you to a religion. No religion healed me or saved me. I'm sharing these things to offer you the same love, hope, and healing I found through a personal relationship with God.

If you haven't said yes to Jesus, will you consider doing that today? I know what happens to a heart that is locked up in emotional chains. I know the devastation and desperation a human soul can feel when every earthly option fails. But I also know the freedom that can *only come* through Jesus, and how miraculously God can intervene when we cry out in brokenness for his mercy.

What do you need Jesus to do for you? Where have you lost hope? Where do you need his touch? You are not alone; Jesus is waiting for you. He is the light that can break through the darkness. He is the one who can overcome the pain. I pray you will make the choice today to open your heart to him. You may not understand what all this means yet, but know this: *you need Jesus and he is enough.* Call on his name, invite him into all the areas of your brokenness. Ask for his forgiveness, and acknowledge your need for him. If you give him your life, you will never be the same.

Wait, I'm a Christian

Christians can also struggle with depression. In fact, Christians tend to hide their innermost feelings more than anyone else, convinced it's not okay to let anyone know they're not okay. We go to church and pretend. But the Bible tells many stories of people who suffered with depression. Many mighty men and women of God—who knew God and walked with him— also knew what it was like to fall into a pit of despair and hopelessness. The good news: God didn't leave them there. In their despair, he cared for them, gave them what they needed, and brought good out of their circumstances. By giving them a new perspective on life, he gave them hope and delivered them out of that pit.

If you're grieving loss, like Naomi,[11] be patient with yourself. Understand depression is a normal part of the grieving process. Allow God to carry you through. Cry out to him in your grief. There is a comfort and healing that can be found when we allow Jesus to grieve with us.[12]

If the depression is brought on by fear and a broken heart, like Elijah, quiet your soul before God and listen for his still, small voice of comfort and direction.[13]

If you spend your days and nights weeping like David,[14] or you are left wondering why your soul is downcast, seek the Lord for answers. Praise him. Praise is uplifting. Put your hope in God, as David did, and you will find renewed strength.[15]

As Christians we are not exempt from pain and hardship. Jesus said, "In this world you will have trouble."[16] But he also told us to take heart because he had overcome the world. Even though we will face many things, in Jesus we have hope and the help we need to overcome and find freedom.

If you are a Christian struggling with despair, here are some things to ponder:

Are you studying God's Word on a regular basis? What do you believe? Do you believe what God says about you? The difference between victory and defeat is our awareness of God's love. Knowing and believing we are loved, no matter what, fills us with hope and joy.

How do you identify God? Our image of God will make us or break us. If we think God is unwilling or unable, we become weak. If we believe God is all powerful, we become empowered.

Are you compromising in your walk with Jesus? Are you comparing yourself with others? Have you fallen into temptation, believing the lies of the enemy over the truth of God? We have an adversary who wants to keep us living under the weight of oppression. Oppression can feel like depression, because it brings on many of the same symptoms; but again, whether we're battling depression or oppression, *Jesus is the heart of the cure.*

As Christians, we have hope for depression the world doesn't understand. But sometimes we fall into despair because we forget that apart from the Savior, there is no better place to find power and comfort in the crisis. No matter how bad things get, God has a way out. He has the power to overcome anything. If you redirect your focus, and remind yourself of God's love, faithfulness, promises, and the power given to you through the Holy Spirit, you can find strength in the fight. If you surround yourself with other Christians who can keep you encouraged and help you build on your relationship with God, you can find inspiration and the motivation to keep going.

Chapter 7

Overcoming Depression

Learning to Live

God can—and wants—to heal and restore every soul struggling with depression. He wants to set each one free, but when seeking his healing, it's important to understand God is sovereign. God is a God of miracles. Nothing is impossible with God. But the way he delivers, and the time frame in which he chooses to release a soul, is completely in his hands. As in my case, he can reach out and heal you in an instant. However, recognize God's primary purpose is to bring wholeness and to bring you close to himself, so he may not heal you the same way he healed me, but be assured, he is able to heal you.

My first step toward healing was allowing myself to be honest with God. Before God could deal with the depression, I had to be authentic with him. That day in the shower, I unleashed the pain I was feeling. I sobbed through every word, but I laid my heart bare. I allowed myself to be vulnerable. I had reached a turning point. Feeling like I had been ground into dust, I had exhausted all other efforts to find healing and had come to the end of myself. I had no one, and nothing left to give but brokenness. So I finally acknowledged and admitted my need for him. In prior prayers, I told God what I wanted him to do, what I thought was needed, and what I expected. But the prayer I prayed that day was a completely different cry for relief and freedom. It was not a mandate nor a way to bargain with God; rather it was an opportunity to proclaim my great need for him. I believe these were the things he had been waiting to hear before unlocking that prison door.

God wants to not only set us free from depression, he wants to set us free from the source of our pain, emotional turmoil, and suffering. Remember, depression has a root. Not all depression is clinical, but the evidence something else is going on. It's a warning, an indicator that underlining problems still need to be dealt with, and only God knows how to expose and reach the deep-seated wounds buried within our souls.

When God released me from the symptoms of depression, it was only the beginning of my journey to freedom. Once I opened my heart to Jesus and asked him to be my Savior, he began a work within my soul that led me to take a deeper look at the wounds I still carried. Through a process of restoration, he touched my heart and mind with his truth and love, which changed the way I thought about things, which in turn stopped the destructive patterns.

Depression is only part of the problem. There is a deeper healing that needs to take place if we are to overcome depression and learn to live free. Only God knows the work and restorative healing that needs to be done. Only he knows how to restore us—mind, body, soul, and spirit.

Getting to the Root

The mercy of being instantly delivered from the symptoms of depression allowed me to breathe again. It felt incredible to be released, finally unshackled from those heavy chains, but a lot of work remained to be done in my heart, mind, and soul. The battle may have been won, but the war wasn't over. Even though the crippling effects of depression were gone, *the wounds ran deep.* The use of alcohol and the physical abuse toward my daughter stopped when the depression lifted, but I still continued to struggle with anger, bouts of rage, fear, and insecurity.

If I was going to be *finally free,* I had to ask God to get to the root of the matter, so I could be free from not only the symptoms of depression, but the cause. I needed to reach a point where I was no longer willing to cover up the emotional roots embedded deep within my soul. In order to find inner healing, I had to go through a process of restoration. I had to trust God, open my heart again, and expose myself to the work that still needed to be done.

As God began to take me through this process, I began to recognize how my emotions had affected me, both positively and negatively, and I learned to never minimize the events of the past even if they seemed trivial. These events had an effect on my soul, and over time these wounds found a way to surface. Because I hadn't dealt with the root of my emotions effectively, I unknowingly allowed them to fester and grow stronger. Since these wounds developed much earlier in life, I thought I had put them behind me. But moving on, or pretending they didn't exist, didn't make them go away. By convincing myself I had gotten over the past, I only covered up the problem.

Prior to the depression surfacing, plenty of indicators told me something was wrong, showing me I had embedded roots of rejection, resentment, bitterness, insecurity, low self-esteem, and shame. And these warning signs became visible through anger or fits of rage every time something happened to trigger a suppressed memory or feeling. In an instant, some seemingly small event would throw me back into a place where old feelings would resurface, bringing with them a tidal wave of emotion.

In order to find freedom, I had to confront the problems I had been covering up. If I didn't, I was merely putting a Band-Aid on a broken bone. Every negative emotion has a root, and these roots don't simply go away. They have to be extracted. Since I hadn't dealt with my emotional roots, I put myself in a state of emotional bondage in which I suffered greatly, and inflicted suffering on others.

Think of it this way: Harmful emotions are like dandelions that grow in your yard. You can mow them over so they no longer appear in the lawn, but a couple of days later, if they haven't been removed from the root, they come back.

In order for the removal procedure to begin, I had to reach a point where I was no longer willing to allow the past hurts to define me. I had to say, "Enough! I'm done! I don't want to feel this way anymore. I don't want to be controlled by anger and rage anymore."

The day I made up my mind was right after I had unexpectedly blown up at two very good friends. At the time I assumed they would understand my bout of anger and be compassionate. I thought they would lovingly put their arms around me in an effort to help me understand why I was so upset. They didn't. Instead, my outburst caught them off guard. They were so stunned for a time they didn't want anything to do with me.

The following day I got on my knees and asked God to get to the root of my anger. "Whatever it takes," I prayed. "Get rid of this anger!" I finally became willing to face the pain instead of running from it—to turn over every wrong and place it in the hands of God's love.

The Journey of Restoration

Getting to the roots was not easy, nor was it automatic. It's human nature to want the cure to be easy. We want being set free to be pain free. But there is no easy way out of emotional bondage. At first it was agonizing as God revealed the embedded roots I had allowed to fester throughout life. As he touched those areas, I found myself, once again, revisiting childhood memories and tender areas of the past. Old feelings of fear and resentment began to resurface which triggered old emotions and revealed scars.

My soul was a tangled mess, a web of emotions keeping me caged. As God worked to unravel the clutter and clean out the debris, I wept more than I did during the depression. Despair and hopelessness did not over take me again, but the pain of my past overwhelmed me to the point that I didn't think I would make it through. I hated having to take a hard look at myself and come face-to-face with what I had done, and the things that had been done to me. But if

I was going to be *finally free*, I had to face the things I didn't want to face. The good news: I didn't have to do it alone.

Restoration Isn't Renovation

Restoration is not renovation. When you renovate something you fix it, but when something is restored, it is put back to its original state. We don't want to merely be fixed, we want to be restored. We don't want to settle for an overhaul—we want to be whole. We don't want to pray, *"God, fix me!"* We want to pray, *"God, restore me!"* Jesus is making all things new.[17] He is restoring what was lost, not fixing it. He is putting everything back to its original state.

Let me illustrate this with a house. Several years ago, my husband and I renovated a one-hundred-year-old historical Victorian gem, although it didn't look like a gem at first. The prior owners of twenty years didn't take care of it at all. So by the time we tried to obtain it, it was considered to be in condemned condition. Though the foundation was good, the city officials wouldn't let us take occupancy. Their plan was to tear the old girl down and lay a parking lot for the growing businesses that surrounded the property. After several meetings, phone calls, and trips to city hall, the city officials finally conceded and allowed us to close on the house.

Once we moved in, we were hit with many unexpected issues. We knew up front the roof leaked and the shutters were barely attached, landscaping was overgrown and partially covered the house, and it desperately needed a paint job. The inside of the house was worse. Dust and cobwebs covered everything, and the stench of death permeated the rooms. Many other hidden problems didn't become obvious until we began the restoration process. The extra work was not something we foresaw, but once these buried flaws were exposed, we were able to deal with them. In the end the house turned out better than we had originally expected.

This is what restoring a life can look like when Jesus (the Master Carpenter) purchases our condemned lives with the sole purpose of restoring our beauty. If instead of tearing ourselves down, and we trust Jesus to restore us, we will be better than we ever hoped we could be. He will deal with the years of neglect, sweep the house clean, and remove the unwanted debris. He will uncover things we either didn't know about or tried to hide. This process can be painful and something we didn't plan on. But when the work is complete, we will be more beautiful than we ever imagined.

While my husband and I worked on that dilapidated old house, we caught the attention of those around us. The neighbors took note, and they too began to refurbish their homes. The local newspaper caught wind of what we were doing and interviewed us a couple of times. Word spread that this old house was getting more than a facelift, and people came from near and far to see the results.

One Christmas, to raise money for the local community, we opened the house for public tours. We were stunned at how many people came, and by the comments they made as they saw each room. Everyone who visited that old house was completely amazed at the fresh appearance of life it reflected. It was better than new—it was restored.

Each of us, in our condemned condition, is like this raggedy old Victorian. But when the Master Carpenter moves in, he begins a process of restorative transformation. Most of us don't realize what's inside, or the damage that has been done until he begins the cleaning and rebuilding process. But if we allow the work to be done, we can become a glorious masterpiece, a work of art others will marvel at.

Don't be afraid of the restoration process. Most of us spend too much time running from everything that makes us feel uncomfortable. Restoration means new life. God wants to get out of you what he put into you. He intends to undo, overdo, and out-do any evil or wrong that has been done to you, but you need to actively cooperate with him in doing the work.

Jesus is a carpenter you can count on to get the job done right. God's greatest work comes when you come to the end of yourself and give him all the broken pieces. So don't run. Open your heart and allow him to begin the construction that will bring wholeness and restoration into your life.

The Beauty of Divine Exchange

As we go through the restoration process, something wonderful happens as Jesus takes our grief and fills us with his joy. He strips away the sackcloth of despair and clothes us in royal garments of praise. He removes our guilt, shame, and disgrace, and gives us hope. He touches our lives with truth and reveals his favor, grace, mercy, and personal love. He takes all the pain and brings healing and freedom to our wounded souls. He takes what was lost, and rebuilds what was stolen.[18]

This exchange sounds beautiful and easy. Who wouldn't want to give up mourning and despair and receive joy and praise? But there may be things you're not ready or willing to face or deal with yet.

It can be difficult to let go of the past and stop harboring bitterness and anger. Sometimes it's easier to hold onto the pain than to forgive someone who harmed us. It's hard to stop blaming ourselves, to stop believing we've blown it, or that we're unworthy, and receive what God is graciously giving us. It's challenging to change the way we've always thought about things, and adopt a new way of thinking and living. To enter freedom, we need to hand over the things that hold us captive. Freedom has a price, but we should never allow the cost to outweigh the result.

I'm not going to lie. At times I struggled greatly, but I got through the fight because I clung to God and worked with him through the process. No matter what was happening or how I felt, I clung to the knowledge that he was exchanging embedded roots for something much sweeter. He was taking pieces of my shattered heart and giving them back to me anew. He was taking all the things I suffered and giving me hope. He was taking my bondage and giving me freedom, taking feelings of death and giving me life.

God wants to do the same for you. Ask him to grant you mercy and the will to fight. Ask him to strengthen your mind, heart, soul, and spirit. If you are ready, ask him to get to the root of the depression—all the pain—and reveal its origin. Make the choice to hand over everything you've been through and trying to hide—all the fears, failures, burdens, bitterness, resentment, insecurity, regrets, and disappointments—and trust God to hand you something beautiful in their place.

The Things that Hold Us Captive

When Jesus sets us free, he releases us from the world's views and the lies of the enemy (the devil). He sets us free from the wrongs done to us, and the afflictions that have nearly destroyed us. When Jesus opens these doors of freedom, his light floods the darkness, illuminating real truth and love. However, whether or not we *remain* free will depend on us.

Sometimes, even after we've been set free, we choose to remain imprisoned. We may momentarily taste the freedom only to put ourselves right back into bondage. Why? Why would anyone allow themselves to be held captive?

Usually we remain in captivity because we don't cooperate with God or allow him to finish the work he has begun. We get stuck in the process, and don't permit him to complete the restoration.

When we identify with the pain, thinking *this is who I am*, it creates a defeated mentality which causes us to settle into the belief that this is a normal way of life. As a result, we become paralyzed by the pain we think defines us. It can be scary to let go, so fear of failure or fear of the unknown can keep us trapped in painful familiarity—a kind of toxic comfort zone—rather than entering an unfamiliar freedom.

We also keep ourselves imprisoned because we refuse to let go of past hurts. We continue to harbor and replay critical attitudes and grievances, allowing them to consume us. Whether consciously or subconsciously, we mentally attempt to get back at someone who harmed us—even though we're the only ones who are suffering from it.

These things create a stronghold. A stronghold is a destructive, recurring, entrenched pattern that can permanently solidify feelings of hopelessness and defeat. It's any lie, attitude, action, or emotion that takes control of our lives over and over again. A stronghold is a yoke; a burden and a hindrance that weighs us down and eventually destroys our lives, if it's not dealt with.

For example, unforgiveness is a stronghold. For some of us, forgiveness is an ugly word. In our minds, forgiving one who has wronged us communicates that the offense the person committed is okay. The abuse is okay. The rape is okay. The betrayal is okay. But it's not okay. No matter what anyone did, it's not okay. If someone harmed you, it's not okay. Forgiving someone from your heart doesn't make what they did okay. Rather, it opens a door that gives *you* an opportunity to be okay.

Forgiveness doesn't right the wrong. It doesn't change the situation or erase it from your memory. Exercising forgiveness—releasing anger, resentment, and the desire for revenge—gives you a lifelong get-out-of-jail-free card, and it keeps you from being thrown back into that jail cell.

According to the parable in Matthew 18:21-35, unless a person forgives from the heart he will be thrown into prison and tortured. If we choose not to forgive from that deep place within our hearts, the pain of resentment and anger continues to grow, gnawing away at us, and tightening the chains that keep us in turmoil. Now that's emotional torture!

Forgiving from the heart is hard. Most of us can achieve an intellectual level of forgiveness on our own. We can say, "I forgive you," and think we mean it, but forgiveness at the heart level is a whole different matter. Only God can help us get to that deep place of forgiveness. Only he can get to the root. And until the issue is dealt with at the heart level by allowing God to get to the root, we will never reach that place of forgiveness where we find healing and freedom for our souls.

Right now you may be thinking: *Wait a minute, I've done nothing wrong! Why should I be the one to forgive?*

What happened may not have been your fault. You didn't ask for the offense, nor did you do anything to provoke it; however, the original hurt someone caused you is only half the problem. If you harbor any bitterness in your heart, it will eat away at you like a cancer and keep you locked up in an emotional prison. So even though none of this may be your fault, forgiveness is an important step to finding freedom and being released from the past.

I understand that when someone has wronged us, hurt us deeply, even hurt someone we love, it's easy to take matters into our own hands and try to bring about vindication, or at least wish evil upon that person. It's human nature to want to lash out, or be resentful and unforgiving. We want the person who hurt us, or hurt our loved one, to suffer. This course of action feels like justice for our suffering. An eye for an eye—right? But the truth is, being unforgiving and vengeful only increases the pain.

Remember, not taking vengeful actions, or forgiving someone for harm they caused, doesn't indicate what they did is okay. Forgiving someone from your heart makes you okay because you are letting go of the pain and putting it into God's hands, giving him the opportunity to vindicate you.[19]

God knows what you've been through. He knows all the pain you've suffered, and he does want to vindicate you. However, in order to receive justification, freedom, and healing, you must first release these things into his hands. Release your desire to get even, and rest in God. Give him the place to act on your behalf. Allow him to give you comfort in your mourning, joy in your grief, and hope in your despair. Let him rebuild what was lost, stolen, and destroyed.

Forgiveness Is the Key to Freedom

As long as I tried to hide my hurt and anger at the physical and emotional abuse inflicted on me as a child, as long as I tried to move forward and not deal with it, hostility and rage grew within my soul. Holding onto all that repressed emotion was like standing beneath a volcano that was about to erupt. The mountain looked pretty from the outside, but inside it was full of hot, molten lava that would one day explode. Repressed emotions eventually surface. When they do, they are like an erupting volcano.

In order to find freedom from all of the hurt and pain from my past, I had to surrender it all to God and forgive. I had to forgive my dad, the kids at school, and all the people who hurt me. Forgiving Dad came about a year after I started going through the restoration process. One morning, as I went about my day, a thought came to mind: *Tell him you love him.* At first I wasn't sure who "he" was. No one in particular came to mind. Then as the thought came to mind a second time, I knew it was my dad.

Still afraid of my dad, I felt nervous to approach him, yet the very next time I saw him I told him I loved him. With tears in his eyes, he hugged me and told me he loved me too. From that time on, he hugged me every chance he got. This was a huge change. Growing up, I could count on one hand the number of times Dad hugged me—now he hugs me all the time. We talk, laugh, play games together, and share thoughts and conversations we never shared before.

I know this sounds far too simple. It may seem impossible for a broken relationship to be repaired so quickly, but what I didn't realize was dad was hurting too. He was no different than me—another wounded soul looking for love. Before that day I never took the time to get to know my father. I didn't know about the things he'd been through; all the things he'd suffered. He never apologized for abusing me. I didn't ask him to. But after hearing his story, I understood my dad in a way I had never understood him before. Understanding his painful past gave me a great deal of insight into mine, and why he treated my brother and me the way he did.

I can't explain what happened the day I told Dad I loved him, but suddenly I was able to forgive him. Not because he deserved my forgiveness or because it now gave me some kind of newfound power over him.

Instead, the love I offered allowed me to open my heart. This type of compassion gave me a release I had never known before.

Forgiving Dad and telling him I loved him was a huge step toward healing. It didn't right the wrong of being abused, but the abuse no longer had as much power over me. Over time, as I continued to go through the restoration process, allowing the divine exchange to take place, I grew stronger. Fear and insecurity didn't hold me captive as they once did, and the repressed anger didn't surface as often. Am I perfect? No. I'm still a work in progress. The difference is now I understand the root source of the pain. I recognize the work God is doing in me, and with his help I am being restored daily.

The One You Need to Forgive

If *you* are the one you need to forgive, I encourage you to take that step. Maybe you feel responsible for the place where you now find yourself. Perhaps the things you've tried to keep quiet are haunting your soul. Life is full of choices, and maybe some of those choices are causing you to feel shame or self-hatred.

I've had many regrets in life, and perhaps the biggest one is how I saw life during the depression. I made choices, said things, did things, and acted in ways that placed a mark of shame on my soul. To embrace freedom, I had to admit my mistakes and forgive myself for all the hurt and pain I had imposed on others.

For example, as I confronted the way I unleashed my repressed anger upon my oldest child, it broke my heart. I lamented how I lashed out at her. And I had to come to a place where I could forgive myself and ask for her forgiveness. She was very young, but the day I shared my heartfelt remorse with her, she immediately began to cry. She threw her arms around my waist and said, "I didn't think you loved me." Thankfully, today she claims not to remember much of the harm I inflicted on her as a child, but I still think those events left a mark on her soul.

To find freedom I had to forgive myself for all the choices I had made, like drinking while my children were around or leaving them unattended while I slept off another dark day of depression. I had to forgive myself for the desire to take my own life and leave my family behind to deal with the loss and aftermath.

Forgiving myself was the hardest part of the restoration process, and far more difficult than forgiving others. Like trying to remove nasty stains in a carpet, my choices lingered in my mind and refused to come out.

It was even harder to believe God forgave me. As a new Christian beginning to go through the restoration process, I was utterly grateful for his healing touch and salvation, but I still hadn't fully grasped God's mercy and unearned grace extended to me through his Son, so I was finding it difficult to let go of my mistakes and accept his forgiveness. Part of me thought God would be like my dad was when I was a child, strict and harsh. Being holy and righteous, how could God offer me anything but condemnation and judgment for the things I had done.

It took time, but my attitude began to change as I studied God's Word. The more I studied and allowed his Word to penetrate my heart, the more I saw the truth of God's heart toward me. I began to realize he wasn't harsh, angry, or displeased with me, he loved me and delighted in me. God's love toward me was unconditional and passionate. He desired to be close to me, and that revelation transformed my heart, mind, and soul. I began to pour myself, my time and energy into my relationship with God, focusing more on God's heart toward me instead of my mistakes. As a result, I began to see God, myself, and those around me differently.

Once I was able to comprehend God's compassionate heart toward me, and internally recognize the reality of his love for me, everything changed. Knowing deep in my heart that God loved me, and gave his Son to die for me[20] and take the punishment for my poor choices, awakened my soul and gave me an opportunity to discover a depth of emotional healing more profound than the original physical healing from depression. Grasping and accepting God's unconditional love and forgiveness toward me became the catalyst for an even greater healing—the healing of my soul.

God's love and forgiveness is beyond my comprehension. The wonderful thing is, I don't have to figure it out—I only need to believe it and receive it. And when I open my heart to embrace that truth, he enables me to love and forgive, even when it is difficult.

Making the Choice to Open Your Heart

If you are feeling despair because of shame. If you find it difficult to forgive yourself for past mistakes, Jesus is here for you. He wants to take every stronghold—every yoke of oppression—and exchange each one of them for his yoke, which is easy and light.[21] With the light of his truth, he wants to expose every lie you are buying into and every attitude keeping you in bondage, and exchange them for the truth of his love for you. He wants to bring healing and freedom to your soul by digging up all the embedded emotional roots, and exchanging each one for something good.

If you and I want to be *finally free*, we need to become vulnerable, be honest with God, and admit our need for him. We need to give him access to the roots we carry by trusting him to take us through a journey of restoration toward wholeness. We can no longer allow our souls to be enslaved by our past, because this captivity feeds and energizes the depression. The process of restoration is not easy, but remember, it will be worth it. Great beauty is found in the divine exchange, as he takes our broken ashes and gives us something beautiful.

Chapter 8

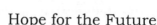

Hope for the Future

Discovering Fresh Purpose and Life

My story, like yours, started on the day I debuted on planet earth. From the moment I took my first breath, my story has been evolving, changing, and growing, and with God's help I've been growing with it. My youth may not have been what I would have chosen. I may have searched for acceptance, happiness, and satisfaction in all the wrong places and suffered from depression as a result. But God used all the suffering, confusion, and emotional pain to reveal a greater purpose—my great need for him. Even though I was indifferent toward him, God never gave up on me. When the symptoms of despair swallowed my life, I ended up finding the only One who could save me, even though I didn't know him personally.

It's remarkable to look back and think about how this God I didn't acknowledge would save someone as messed up as me. At my lowest point, when I had exhausted all other options and efforts to find relief, he reached into the turmoil of my personal madness and set me free. Not only that, with his mercy came a miraculous and powerful testimony of hope, of love and deliverance, of healing power, and his unfathomable grace.

In the midst of it all, something extraordinary began to dawn on me: *God had a specific plan for my life.* Even with all my planning, hopes, and dreams for the future, he had something better. And through the course of my life, he deliberately unveiled that plan. Never in my wildest dreams would I have guessed God would take what I had been through and use it as a light in dark places. For more than two decades, God has taken my story and given me countless opportunities to share his amazing grace on national television and radio; in books, blogs, and magazine articles; and before various groups, churches, and women's organizations. I don't share these things to boast or brag, but to offer you hope. Testimonies have a way of touching the untouchable, and opening a door for restoration and optimism that may not have been there before.

Purpose Can Be Found in the Pain

We all have hopes and dreams. We all long for a sense of purpose, and there is no greater purpose than our God-ordained destiny. No matter what we go through, no matter what is causing the depression, as we heal, God can take everything and use it as a message of hope to inspire and challenge others.

In God's hands, pain has a purpose. We may not be able to make sense of the things we go through, but every trial that hits our lives is bursting with divine determination to bring forth something good.

I like to call it *Nightmare to Ministry.* Nightmare to Ministry happens when God uses the worst part of our lives in order to bring out the best part of us. In the midst of our circumstances, at the height of our worst nightmare, God says, *"I choose you. Not in spite of your past, but because of it."* God wants to take our worst nightmare, redeem it, restore it, and use it for good— not only for His glory, but for the encouragement and support of others who are still suffering.

Never give up the fight for freedom. God wants to redeem your past and give you a powerful testimony— to give you a hope and a future. A new song waits for you, a song that boldly sings of his love and mercy— one you can share with those he places around you. Ask God to help you tap into the plan and purpose he has for you. There is a light waiting to break through the darkness, and when it does, your life will burst with fresh meaning.

Right now you may be feeling unfit to help anyone. You may be thinking; *I don't have it in me.* I understand. At the height of the depression, the last thing I would have wanted to do was help someone else, especially someone with depression. I was suffering. I was the one who needed help. The darkness blinded me to any sort of purpose. I couldn't see how anything good could come from my present condition.

When we're going through difficult situations, the pain is often more than we can bear. We don't have the strength and energy to help others, because all we can think about is how urgently we need help. We aren't capable of seeing or understanding there is purpose in the madness. We can't grasp the possibility that one day our pain could be someone else's miracle.

I am living proof God can and will redeem a harmful past in order to give someone else hope for the future. But I wasn't completely whole when God began to use me. When I started sharing my testimony publicly, I had only begun to go through the restoration process. I didn't have all the answers. I didn't understand all of what God wanted to do with my testimony, I just knew I had one and was invited to tell it.

Dear One, God is not finished with you. He is not surprised or caught off guard by what you are going through. He has not abandoned you to the darkness. You may still be struggling, but the depression is not the end. It's a chance for a new beginning. The depression will not last forever. In his time and in his own way, God will deliver you and give you a powerful testimony. And, when he does, share your story. Tell others what he has done for you. You don't need to be a public speaker. You don't need to be perfect; you just need to be willing. Just trust God to use whatever you've been through to touch and change the lives of others.

A Glorious Future Filled with Hope

One of the reasons I like to talk about the depression and the pain of the past is because every time I do, another piece of my heart is rebuilt. Every time I share my story, I am reminded of God's goodness and I am renewed. And when he takes my story and everything I've been through and changes another life, I am blessed.

About six months after God touched my life, I was invited to speak at a local church during a MOPS Appreciation Night. Approximately three hundred women and their spouses listened as I recounted what happened. Standing up front felt surreal. Even though the words came out of my mouth with ease, I felt more like a spectator than a participant. When I was finished, I quickly handed the microphone to the woman in charge, only to realize she was crying. Without taking the microphone, she stood up, buried her face in my shoulder and wept. Then I noticed another woman walking toward us, and she was crying. As the three of us huddled together up front, I began to look out at the audience. Almost everyone was crying.

What did I say? was the question reverberating in my heart. God touched so many lives that night but none more powerfully than Angie.

Angie approached me afterward and began to share how God used my story to speak into her life. Her past year had been devastating. Within twelve short months she had lost her husband, her only son, her mother, and her dog. But hearing my testimony and the power of God's instant healing gave her hope. She no longer felt helpless and desperate—she now felt the love of a God whom she thought had forsaken her.

The ironic thing was Angie didn't know the church I was speaking at existed. It wasn't a small church, but it was out on a country road, away from the city. She told me she was so depressed and lonely that she was on her way to commit suicide by driving her car off a bridge. As she drove by the church, there were so many cars in the parking lot that curiosity took over, and she decided to come in. Angie had no idea what the event was or what she was about to hear, but God directed her path. Once inside, she heard me talking up front and was drawn by my story.

Angie didn't commit suicide that night. In fact, we wrote to each other for a long time afterward. Therefore, it is for the Angies of this world that I am grateful for the depression, the suffering, the heartache of a painful past—everything I endured in order to offer encouragement to another hurting soul. This is not to say I'm happy I went through depression, but now I see there was a bigger plan at work.

I know suffering is not fun, and there is still a part of me that would never want to go back. But if you asked me today if I would be willing to suffer the effects of depression all over again, I would say, "In a heartbeat!" When I consider what God took me through, and how he used that season of my life to help others find freedom and healing, then, "yes," I would do it all again. Knowing what I know now, and how God would take the ashes of my suffering to create something beautiful, I would do it all over again. I would endure every debilitating moment knowing that I had a future formed by the grace of God to bring hope to others.

Learn to Tie Rags

Perhaps what I am saying is giving you a fresh perspective on your own situation. Or maybe not. Maybe the chains of depression are gripping you so tight you have lost hope of ever getting free. Don't give up. God sees where you are. He wants to touch your life and reveal the plan and purpose he has for you. Everything may feel like it's falling apart, but don't let the circumstances of life extinguish your hope. What you're going through is the very thing God can use to touch the life of another.

On the other hand, maybe you've already been set free, but you never allowed God to use your suffering for his purposes. Maybe the thought of going back to the well causes you to shutter. Or you don't think you can tie rags together in order to help those who have fallen, like Ebed-Melek and the other men who set Jeremiah free. Once you are free from that place of darkness it's difficult to return. But listen, you will not be *finally free* until God takes your pain, transforms it, and uses it. Until you offer yourself to others with the comfort he has given you,[22] a part of you will remain unhealed.

Freedom doesn't come because our circumstances have changed. Freedom comes when we are no longer afraid to face the things that hurt us. Freedom enables us to embrace the past instead of running from it. Freedom helps us go back, analyze what we went through, and offer hope to someone else.

The men and women I know who share their stories have something in their past that motivates their future. For example, I know a gal who wrote a book called *Damaged Goods: Learning to Dream Again.*[23] In her book she shares her traumatic past of physical and sexual abuse, and her struggle to find love and acceptance. Her heart-rending trials led her to depression and seven suicide attempts until God redeemed her past in order to give her a powerful present and future. Now through her book and speaking, she shares with audiences all over the world, helping them to let go of their painful past by teaching them to dream again.

My friend Sheryl Griffin wrote a book called *A Scarlet Cord of Hope: My Journey Through Guilt, Shame, and Fear to Hope.*[24] Through her story, Sheryl tells about her painful past with alcoholic parents, an abusive first marriage, and abortion. The effects of these events, coupled with the choices she made throughout life, brought on overwhelming feelings of shame, which caused severe panic and anxiety attacks. But in the midst of her suffering, God showed Sheryl how to put together the puzzle pieces of her life by helping her grasp his cord of hope. Now Sheryl shares her story openly, wanting others to know they are not alone, and that they do not have to be entangled by the emotional cords of guilt, fear, and shame.

Another precious woman I know has been battling cancer, alongside her two sons, for the past twenty-six years. Between the three of them, they have been diagnosed many times, undergone years of chemotherapy and numerous surgeries to remove cancerous nodes, including amputation. Her older son, Christopher, continues to fight for his life after recently undergoing surgery to replace the bones in his infected arm and leg. Yet throughout their journey, she remains a constant advocate for her sons, encouraging them and lifting their spirits. "Together," Teresa says, "we learned to face every challenge with an open heart, to live joyfully, and to laugh and smile as much as possible. We have learned that life here on earth is not the end, and each moment is a gift."

During his college years, Laurence Tumpag became homeless. Today he is off the streets and employed as a social worker, helping the struggling children and families of his community. "I am grateful," he says, "for the days of poverty." His experience of living in destitution has not only become a personal banner of courage and self-determination, but also an incredible opportunity to understand and assist others who are hurting as he once did.

We don't share our stories for applause, fame, money, or book sales. We share our stories of what God has done in order to offer people hope, so they too can find the love, power, grace, mercy, and hope we have found through the heart of a redeeming Savior.

The Only Pure Joy is in Jesus

I don't pretend to understand why certain things happen, or why God allows such deep pain to touch our lives, but when I don't understand, I rest on who I know God is and trust him to bring something good from the pain. No matter what happens, I know in the core of my soul that God loves me and has a plan. It's that conscious awareness of God's heart that gives me joy in the pain and hope for tomorrow. I have personally experienced God's power and personal love. He has become more real to me than any human being standing next to me. And I know, without doubt, he can take every bad situation and exchange it for something good. I know he is a Redeemer who restores what was lost or stolen. I know he is the source of life that gives hope for today and tomorrow.

Don't let incorrect information or a bad church experience hold you back from reaching out and knowing the only One who can give you the healing you so desperately need.

At one time I was convinced living a happy and exciting life was found in people, money, places, and things. It's been nearly four decades since I first carried those attitudes, and over the years I've done a lot of living and made a lot of mistakes. Yet I've learned a great deal and have overcome much. This is not to say I have it all figured out, but what my experiences have taught me is the truth behind what the speaker shared that day at the MOPS meeting. Everyone goes through terrible heartache, suffering, grief, regret, and disillusionment. Life will disappoint us and throw us a few curve balls. But in the heart of her message, was an answer to all the heartache and troubles of this world: *The only pure joy is in Jesus.*

Is everything perfect since I was healed and gave my life to Jesus? No, I still have bad days and painful times when I feel sad or discouraged, fearful, or even angry. But instead of allowing those feelings to control me or throw me back into despair, I remember what he has done, and the great love he has shown me. That is what fills me with joy and gives me the strength to overcome whatever I am going through.

Prior to knowing Jesus, I thought I understood what it meant to be happy and to have joy. I realize now I wasted too much time worrying about what I had and what I didn't have. These false pursuits only distracted me from the truth, robbed me of joy, and could never fill the void in my soul. No more! I will no longer put my life in the hands of empty promises. I want joy—pure joy—not some fleeting feeling of elation that is here one day and gone the next. I want a deep, inner joy that brings stability to my mind and peace to my soul, even when life is falling apart. I want a joy that will break through the darkest days, lift my spirits, and fill me with faith. And the only way I know to experience that kind of joy is through Jesus. When I trust in his promises, I find hope in his plan and rest for my soul. When I'm consumed with Jesus, those are the days, I am *finally free*!

Special Addition

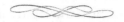

When Someone You Love Is Suffering
Knowing Both Sides of the Well

While writing *Finally Free*, I was approached by many people who have a friend or loved one suffering with depression. They were looking for answers because they didn't know how to manage the depression or help the one they love. I understand what it feels like to be trapped in the well of depression and what it's like to stand on the outside of that well, watching someone I love struggle. Both situations can bring feelings of helplessness and hopelessness.

Seven years after my bout with depression, my husband fell into depression. There were warning signs telling us his world was about to cave in. But, as he had done with me, he ignored those symptoms, hoping everything would get better. It didn't. I recognized something was wrong but remained silent. As the warning signs intensified, I must admit at first I felt frightened. At that point I had been sharing my testimony publicly for some time. But it's one thing to share my story, point to Jesus, and encourage others in their struggles. It's quite another to live with someone who is depressed. Once my husband was clinically diagnosed, I quickly moved past any fear of facing that deep well again and dug in, willing to walk out this journey with him each step of the way.

Unlike me, my husband ended up being hospitalized, where he was immediately prescribed medication. Four months on anti-depressants helped with the symptoms, but they did not make him well. Fearful he would become dependent on the medication, and without the doctor's consent, my husband decided to take himself off of his prescription. This decision caused his condition to worsen. For the next three months his body went through withdrawal. It was a roller coaster ride of emotional highs and lows that at times sent his life spinning out of control.

As I mentioned earlier, many things can cause depression, but not all depression is clinical, and not all depression is mental illness. Some forms of depression *may* require medical diagnosis and treatment. But understand this: although medication may help relieve symptoms, medication *will not cure* depression. I am not advocating medication as a way to find release from depression, nor am I telling you not to seek medical advice. These are decisions you and your loved one will need to consider, and I pray you make these choices under the direction and wisdom of God.

My purpose in sharing my husband's experience with medication is to inform you of the potential risks. Anti-depressants affect the brain. Before beginning any medical treatment for depression, have your loved one analyzed. If you do make the choice to place your loved one on medication under a doctor's care, please stay in close contact with the doctor. Make sure the doctor instructs you before stopping any prescription drugs. The effects of abruptly stopping anti-depressants are not pretty and can be dangerous.

Once the anti-depressants were out of his system, my husband did begin to improve emotionally and physically. In time, with counseling, lots of love, and encouragement, he got better and was able to move forward.

From One Caregiver to Another

When a loved one suffers from depression, your support and encouragement can play an important role in his or her recovery. However, depression can also drain you and wear you down if you do not take care of yourself in the process.

As you watch your loved one struggle, it may cause you to feel any number of emotions, including frustration, anger, helplessness and fear, or guilt and sadness. All these feelings are normal, so do not become discouraged. It is not easy dealing with another person's depression, so it's vital you continue to take care of yourself. It is not selfish to think of your own needs and emotional health—it's a necessity! You cannot help someone else if you are run down, overwhelmed, and exhausted.

My husband's depression lasted a year, and through it all, I stood by him. I encouraged him, prayed with him, and drove him to every counseling appointment. During the few days of his initial hospital stay, I was there for every possible minute of visitation. I listened, smiled when he talked, and held him while he cried. Once he was back home, we went for long walks in the park in order to get him out of the house. For a change of pace, we took our family on a mini-vacation, and it helped.

As he gradually progressed, I had to be consistent in my role as a caregiver. I had to be a good listener. I couldn't brush off the way he was feeling, or only offer a few kind words of encouragement. That wouldn't help. I also knew I couldn't save my husband. His release from depression wasn't in my hands, so I never tried to take on any heroics. My primary role was to listen, love him, and be there when he needed me.

During this dark time, to keep myself encouraged and stable, I joined a Bible study, stayed connected to other Christians, and focused on Jesus. Since I clung to the Savior as my sole source of support, I never lost hope. Plus, my spiritual relationship with Jesus soared to new heights of love and trust. In the midst of it all, I believed God could and would free my husband, if he would open his heart and respond to Jesus. This confident resolve gave me the strength to encourage my husband to be optimistic, and reassure him that God loved him and longed to give him a way out.

My husband didn't experience the instant deliverance I did, but God healed him nonetheless. Trusting God is critical, and as I said in Chapter Seven, God is sovereign. We're all different, and the way he chooses to heal is completely in his hands. My husband learned to trust God one day at a time as he surrendered more and more of his life to Jesus. Today he knows Jesus as both his Savior and his healer.

On this journey toward emotional freedom with your loved one, I would like to offer you some practical tips—a list of do's and don'ts—when helping someone you love. Some of these suggestions may not work for everyone, but hopefully they will offer you support and give you a more effective approach. I am not a doctor. I cannot offer professional or medical advice. But I can offer recommendations based on my personal experience and what I learned in dealing with my husband's struggle.

- **Do not underestimate the seriousness of depression** and assume your loved one will be fine. Depression cripples the mind, heart, soul, and spirit. Therefore, do not tell someone to "just get over it." Telling someone, "It's all in your head," or "Look on the bright side," or "Snap out of it," will not help. Your loved one cannot just "snap out of it" by choosing to get better.

- **What you can say that may help is,** "You are not alone, I'm here for you." "I don't understand how you feel, but I care about you and want to help." "You are important to me. Tell me how I can help."

- **Do not ask generalized questions,** such as, "How are you feeling?" or "Is everything ok?" These questions are too vague and will only lead to vague responses.

- **Do ask open-ended questions** that will require more than a one-word response. Instead ask, "When did you begin feeling this way?" "Did something happen that caused you to feel this way?" "How can I best support you right now?"

- **Avoid common communication barriers.** Don't say, "You're not thinking clearly." "If you'll calm down, I'll listen to you." "Stop talking nonsense, get that thought out of your head," "Why don't you..." or "Why did you do that?" These types of statements tend to shutdown communication.

- **Be supportive.** When talking with someone about the depression, remember it's about offering encouragement and hope.

- **Be a good listener.** Be patient, listen attentively, and when responding don't judge or criticize how the person feels. Do not try to fix your loved one. Being a compassionate listener is far more important than giving good advice. So often just having someone to talk to about how they feel can be a wonderful encouragement and help battle the depression.

- **Be transparent.** If you've never experienced depression, do not say you understand. Just empathize. Do share a time when you struggled emotionally. Your transparency can help. Don't expect or force a response. It's risky to lay the soul bare and be exposed. Be patient. Affirm that you are there for them, and when they choose to talk, you will be eager to listen.

* **Have a physical.** It's important to treat the whole person. If it has been a while since their last physical, schedule an appointment with the doctor. Have blood work done to make sure there are no underlining physical issues, like thyroid imbalance, which can lead to depression.

* **Watch for changes in behavior.** Take note if your loved one exhibits any changes in sleep patterns, loss or gain of appetite, withdraws from friends or activities they once enjoyed, turns to drugs or alcohol, or anything else that is completely out of the norm.

* **Help your loved one obtain a healthy lifestyle.** Vitamin deficiency, poor diet, and lack of exercise, all play a role, so help your loved one eat a healthy diet and get the exercise they need. Avoid caffeine, sugar, processed foods, and greasy foods, which can increase levels of anxiety and depression.

* **Do not take it personally.** Depression makes it difficult to connect on an emotional level with anyone, even the people they love most. Depressed people often withdraw or say hurtful things and lash out in anger. Your loved one may at times push you away or say things that are cruel. This behavior stems

from an involuntary and irrational reaction; it's a symptom of the depression. Be understanding and try not to take it personally.

- **Get them out of the house.** Depressed people have a difficult time being around others and are prone to withdraw. Isolation can make the depression worse. They will need help and encouragement to get beyond this place of isolation. Regularly invite, even push, your loved one to join you for a walk, dinner out, or someplace fun. Tap into what they loved to do prior to the depression symptoms.

- **Smile.** A happy face, bright attitude, and cheerful actions may help to lift a downcast spirit.

- **Know when to get help.** People who become suicidal have come to a place of hopelessness. Sometimes your loved one will start showing signs before verbalizing their thoughts about being suicidal or taking action. QPR (Question, Persuade, Refer) provides innovative, practical, and proven suicide prevention training. Learn more at www.qprinstitute.com

- **If the depression worsens,** or you feel there is an impending risk of suicide, do not panic and seek help immediately. Call the National Suicide Hotline: 1-800-273-8255, or call your local prevention hotline number.

- **Seek support.** Depression is overwhelming for everyone involved. Caregivers need to stay emotionally healthy. Join a support group or a Bible study. Talk to a counselor, pastor, or confide in a trusted friend who can help you get through this difficult time. You do not need to go into detail or betray a confidence; rather, focus on your emotional needs.

- **Hold onto faith.** Stay focused on Jesus so you do not lose hope. God is a Healer and Restorer. Your loved one is encouraged best when those around them remain hopeful. Remain connected to God through his Word and the Holy Spirit. Assure your loved one often of God's love for them personally. Read Scripture aloud daily. Play worship music in your home to help keep a positive atmosphere.

- **Seek God in worship.** Draw from his divine power to give you strength, perspective, peace, and joy.

- **Pray for God's help.** Everyone involved will need God's divine intervention. Prayer is the only way to access the inner fortification and wisdom you will need to stand strong in the battle against depression.

Words of Hope

To help you and your loved one find encouragement, below is a list of Scripture verses. These *Words of Hope* are meant to support and uplift you both during this time.

Why are you downcast, O my soul? Why so disturbed within me? Put your hope in God, for I will yet praise Him, my Savior and my God
–Psalm 42:5

In this world you will have trouble. But take heart! I have overcome the world
–John 16:33b

Cast all your anxiety upon him because he cares for you
–1 Peter 5:7

Come to me, all you who are weary and burdened, and I will give you rest. Take my yoke upon you and learn from me, for I am gentle and humble in heart, and you will find rest for your souls
–Matthew 11:28-29

So do not fear, for I am with you; do not be dismayed,
for I am your God. I will strengthen you and help you;
I will uphold you with my righteous right hand
–Isaiah 41:10

...weeping may remain for a night, but rejoicing comes
in the morning
–Psalm 30:5b

I will build you up again and you will be
rebuilt....Again you will take up your tambourines and
go out to dance with the joyful
–Jeremiah 31:4

It is for freedom that Christ has set us free. Stand
firm, then, and do not let yourselves be burdened
again by a yoke of slavery
–Galatians 5:1

So if the Son sets you free, you will be free indeed
–John 8:36

□

...those who hope in the LORD will renew their
strength
–Isaiah 40:31

The LORD is close to the brokenhearted and saves
those who are crushed in spirit
–Psalm 34:18

You will keep in perfect peace him whose mind is
steadfast, because he trusts in you
–Isaiah 26:3

Praise the LORD, O my soul, and forget not all his
benefits—who forgives all your sins and heals all your
diseases, who redeems your life from the pit and
crowns you with love and compassion
–Psalm 103:2-4

You are my lamp, O LORD; the LORD turns my
darkness into light
–2 Samuel 22:29

The people walking in darkness have seen a great
light; on those living in the land of the shadow of
death a light has dawned
–Isaiah 9:2

"For I know the plans I have for you," declares the
LORD, "plans to prosper you and not to harm you,
plans to give you hope and a future"
–Jeremiah 29:11

Trust in the LORD with all your heart and lean not on
your own understanding; in all your ways
acknowledge him, and he will make your paths
straight
–Proverbs 3:5-6

...the LORD has anointed me to preach good news to
the poor. He has sent me to bind up the
brokenhearted, to proclaim freedom for the captives
and release from darkness for the prisoners
–Isaiah 61:1

The ransomed of the LORD will return. They will enter
Zion with singing; everlasting joy will crown their
heads. Gladness and joy will overtake them, and
sorrow and sighing will flee away
–Isaiah 51:11

Praise be to the God and Father of our Lord Jesus
Christ, the Father of compassion and the God of all
comfort, who comforts us in all our troubles, so that
we can comfort those in any trouble with the comfort
we ourselves have received from God
–2 Corinthians 1:3-4

The LORD is a refuge for the oppressed, a stronghold
in times of trouble. Those who know your name will
trust in you, for you, LORD, have never forsaken those
who seek you
–Psalm 9:9-10

God has delivered me from going down to the pit, and I
shall live to enjoy the light of life
–Job 33:28

"Because he loves me," says the LORD, "I will rescue
him; I will protect him, for he acknowledges my name.
He will call upon me, and I will answer him; I will be
with him in trouble. With long life will I satisfy him
and show him my salvation"
–Psalm 91:14-16

A Biblical Perspective On Depression

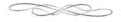

We've talked a lot about depression, but what does the Bible say about it? With the exception of a few translations, the Bible doesn't use the word "depression." However, it often uses comparable words or phrases, such as "downcast," "oppressed, "brokenhearted," "gloom," "darkness," misery," "despair," "mourning," and "going down into the pit," among others. As mentioned in Chapter Six, the Bible tells of many stories of godly men and women of faith who struggled through times of hopelessness and despair.

After great success, Elijah became discouraged, weary, and afraid. In a moment of weakness, he cried out to God, *"I have had enough LORD," he said. "Take my life; I am no better than my ancestors"* (1Kings 19:4).

Jeremiah, known as the weeping prophet because of all he endured, displayed great spiritual faith and strength; yet he struggled with loneliness, feelings of defeat, rejection, insecurity, and failure. He even went so far as to say, *"Cursed be the day I was born! Why did I ever come out of the womb to see trouble and sorrow and to end my days in shame"* (Jeremiah 20:14a,18)?

Job, a righteous man of God, suffered great loss, devastation, and physical illness. Although Job stayed true to God throughout his life, he still struggled intensely through the trenches of pain and loss. Among his confessions was, *"I have no peace, no quietness; I have no rest, but only turmoil"* (Job 3:26).

At the loss of her husband and both sons, Naomi became so depressed she couldn't see anything but the darkness. The pain within her was so great, her only response was to blame God. *"Don't call me Naomi,"* she told them. *"Call me Mara, because the Almighty has made my life very bitter. I went away full, but the LORD has brought me back empty. Why call me Naomi? The LORD has afflicted me; the Almighty has brought misfortune upon me"* (Ruth 1:20-21).

Even though they struggled emotionally, spiritually, and physically; despaired of life, lost hope, and even blamed God, he never abandoned them. He heard their cries, strengthened them, encouraged them, delivered them, restored them, and even changed the course of their lives.

But what about our own struggles with depression? What can we do? What will God do? How can we overcome and find freedom from a biblical standpoint? In this final section, let's consider some verses so we can reflect on depression from a biblical perspective—its causes and its cures.

Cause: Lack of Meaning

"I denied myself nothing my eyes desired; I refused my heart no pleasure. My heart took delight in all my work, and this was the reward for all my labor. Yet when I surveyed all that my hands had done and what I had toiled to achieve, everything was meaningless, a

chasing after the wind; nothing was gained under the sun" (Ecclesiastes 2:10-11).

- At the end of his life, King Solomon was inspired to write the book of Ecclesiastes. Solomon was the wisest and richest king who ever lived, yet his wealth and wisdom didn't make him happy. As he surveyed everything he had achieved, he felt depressed because everything felt meaningless—a chasing after the wind. Solomon had a great life filled with prosperity, fame, and honor, yet none of it brought him satisfaction (see also Ecclesiastes 2:17-23; Ecclesiastes 4:1).

Cure: Where do we find a sense of true purpose?

"For in him we live and move and have our being" (Acts 17:28).

"For we are God's handiwork, created in Christ Jesus to do good works, which God prepared in advance for us to do" (Ephesians 2:10).

- Our purpose doesn't come from what we do. Our purpose comes from our identity in Jesus and what he has done for us. If we do not rest in the knowledge that we are created by him, for him, and for his good pleasure, we will struggle to find contentment and meaning in life (see Colossians 1:15-17). The way to overcome a lack of meaning is to intimately know the One to whom you belong (also see 1 Corinthians 3:23).

Cause: Comparison

"And I saw that all labor and all achievement spring from man's envy of his neighbor. This too is meaningless, a chasing after the wind" (Ecclesiastes 4:4).

- In Ecclesiastes 4:4, Solomon expressed how we often toil in order to impress others or to be like someone else. Comparison always ends badly. We either feel falsely proud of being superior, or we feel falsely discouraged because we feel inferior. It's a trap many of us fall into because we seek acceptance or approval. Laboring with wrong motives can cause us to feel drained, exhausted, dissatisfied, and discontented, which in turn leads to depression.

Cure: How can we defeat feelings of comparison, disappointment, and discouragement, and find satisfaction?

"Trust in the LORD and do good.... Delight yourself in the LORD, and he will give you the desires of your heart" (Psalm 37:3-4).

- When we try to find our self-worth in wealth and riches or success and power, instead of finding our worth in God, we rob ourselves of true joy in life. The only way to overcome dissatisfaction and be content with who we are and what we have is to enjoy God and trust him, to do good to others and not compete. Satisfaction in life is a gift from God. Without him, we are unable to find true enjoyment and contentment in life (see Ecclesiastes 2:24-26; 5:18-20).

Cause: Sin and Rebellion

"Some sat in darkness and deepest gloom, prisoners suffering in iron chains, for they had rebelled against the words of God and despised the counsel of the Most High" (Psalm 107:10-11).

- Continuing to live a sinful lifestyle and refusing to repent, not only separates us from God's fellowship, but it can also bring depression into our lives.

Cure: What can we do to overcome depression brought on by sin and rebellion?

"Then they cried out to the Lord in their trouble, and he saved them from their distress. He brought them out of darkness and the deepest gloom and broke away their chains" (Psalm 107:13-14).

- When those who sat in darkness cried out to God in repentance, he saved them. Even though they were foolish and rebelled against him (Psalm 107:17), he sent forth his word and healed them (Psalm 107:20). In the distress of sin and rebellion, if we turn back to God and cry out in remorse, he will save us and heal us. The affliction of depression is no match for a redeeming God who hears our broken and contrite hearts (see Psalm 51:17).

Cause: Spiritual Attack and Oppression

"For the enemy has pursued and persecuted my soul, he has crushed my life down to the ground; he has made me to dwell in dark places as those who

have been long dead. Therefore, is my spirit overwhelmed and faints within me [wrapped in gloom]; my heart within my bosom grows numb" (Psalm 143:3-4, AMP).

- Some Christians may tell you that all depression and anxiety are purely spiritual battles to be fearlessly conquered with more faith, more Bible reading, and more time spent in prayer. But as we've seen thus far, not all depression is spiritual attack. However, at times, a spirit of despair can come upon us (see Isaiah 61:3). The enemy of our souls (the devil), wants us to live oppressed, weighed down in defeat, riddled by lies, and without hope. So if we give the enemy an open door, he can cast on us a spirit of heaviness. That spirit can cause us to feel depressed and full of hopelessness, even when God is at work in our lives.

Cure: How can we overcome depression brought on by spiritual attack?

"...be strong in the Lord and in his mighty power" (Ephesians 6:10).

- According to 1 John 4:4, we are overcomers because the One who is in us is greater than the one who is doing the attacking. Plus, God has given us weapons that have divine power and authority to demolish strongholds, annihilate false arguments and deception, and take captive every thought and make it submit to God's truth (see 2 Corinthians 10:4-5). If you are in Christ, then Christ is in you, and he has given you the power to overcome every lie that plagues you, and the enemy who tries to defeat you. You may feel downcast. You may want to give up, but God is with you. Open your mouth and proclaim God's truth aloud. Ask him to take from you that spirit of despair and give you a garment of praise. Call on the name of Jesus and he will be your strength in the battle.

Cause: Unforgiveness

"But if you refuse to forgive others, your Father will not forgive your sins" (Matthew 6:15, NLT).

- In Matthew 18:21-35, Jesus told Peter a story about the unmerciful servant who refused to forgive. As a result of his unforgiveness, he was thrown into prison and tortured. When we harbor resentment and anger toward another, those harmful emotions can throw us into an emotional prison of gloom and misery.

Cure: How can we overcome depression brought on by unforgiveness?

"If you, O LORD, kept a record of sins, O Lord, who could stand? But with you there is forgiveness; therefore, you are feared. I wait for the LORD, my soul waits, and in his word I put my hope" (Psalm 130:3-5).

- Forgiveness is God's unmerited grace toward us. Even while we were still sinners, Christ died for us (see Romans 5:8). If you are finding it difficult to forgive someone, or even forgive yourself, take a deep breath and ask for an awareness of God's forgiveness toward you to wash over you. Recognizing the mercy of God's forgiveness toward us helps us forgive, so we can be set free from the emotional torment.

Cause: Harmful Thoughts and Words

"But whatever comes out of the mouth comes from the heart, and this is what makes a man unclean and defiles [him]" (Matthew 15:18, AMP).

- Our thoughts, attitudes, and words can be toxic to our souls. We can bring depression into our lives by what we think about and by what we speak. The tongue has power. With it we can speak life or we can speak death, but either way we will eat its fruit (see Proverbs 18:20-21).

Cure: When our words and attitudes have us feeling downcast, what can we do?

"Finally, brothers and sisters, whatever is true, whatever is noble, whatever is right, whatever is pure, whatever is lovely, whatever is admirable—if anything is excellent or praiseworthy—think about such things" (Philippians 4:8).

"Do not let any unwholesome talk come out of your mouths, but only what is helpful for building others up according to their needs, that it may benefit those who listen" (Ephesians 4:29).

- When our thoughts and words fill us with despair, we still have hope. No matter how many mistakes we've made with our thoughts and words, God can redeem and restore. Let us remain in him (see John 15:7), and let his word dwell richly in us (see Colossians 3:16). Let us meditate on God's Word day and night (see Psalm 1:2) until our thoughts become consumed with his truth. When our thoughts are filled with him, our mouths will begin speaking the very words of God (see 1 Peter 4:11).

Cause: Worry and Anxiety

"Anxiety in a person's heart weighs him down, but an encouraging word brings him joy" Proverbs 12:25, NET).

- In Psalm 6, King David was overwhelmed, full of fear, anxiety, anguish, and despair, because he was worried about his life and what would happen if... Many of us fall into the pit of depression because we worry ourselves sick. We fret about life—our health, our finances and jobs, our families, and our future.

Cure: How can we overcome worry and anxiety?

"So then, banish anxiety from your heart and cast off the troubles of your body..." (Ecclesiastes 11:10).

"Do not be anxious about anything, but in everything, by prayer and petition, with thanksgiving, present your requests to God" (Philippians 4:6).

- David wept and despaired for so long he became weak and frail, but he never gave up hope. In his weakness and great distress, he cried out to God (see Psalm 6:4, 9). He trusted in God's unfailing love to deliver him. We can do the same. In Matthew 6:25, Jesus tells us not to worry about our lives, but to seek first God's kingdom and his righteousness, and he will take care of our needs (v. 6:33).

Cause: Not Having an Eternal Perspective

"My soul has been rejected from peace; I have forgotten happiness. So I say, "My strength has perished, and so has my hope from the LORD" (Lamentations 3:17-18, NASB).

"Sin will be rampant everywhere, and the love of many will grow cold" (Matthew 24:12, NLT).

- Is this not what we see happening today? Without an eternal perspective, our souls can grow weary and fill with despair at the events taking place in the world. But no matter what happens in life or what we witness, it is all temporary. As Paul said, "I consider that our present sufferings are not worth comparing with the glory that will be revealed in us" (Romans 8:18). Our true citizenship is in heaven, not here on earth (see Philippians 3:20). Our hope is not in this world, but in the living hope given to us through Christ Jesus, and kept for us as an imperishable inheritance in heaven (see 1 Peter 1:3-5).

Cure: How can we shift our focus from worldly events to an eternal hope?

"Since, then, you have been raised with Christ, set your hearts on things above, where Christ is seated at the right hand of God. Set your minds on things above, not on earthly things" (Colossians 3:1-2).

"... prepare your minds for action, keep sober in spirit, fix your hope completely on the grace to be brought to you at the revelation of Jesus Christ" (1Peter 1:13, NASB).

"Rejoice in our confident hope. Be patient in trouble, and keep on praying" (Romans 12:12, NLT).

- There will be a day when God will wipe away every tear from our eyes, and death shall be no more, neither shall there be mourning, nor crying, nor pain, for the former things have passed away (see Revelation 21:4). Until then keep watch (see Matthew 24:42-44), be patient; strengthen your heart, for the coming of the Lord is near (see James 5:8-9, NASB).

In Times of Weakness, God Is our Strength

"Why are you downcast, O my soul? Why so disturbed within me? Put your hope in God, for I will yet praise him, my Savior and my God" (Psalm 42:5).

In the midst of depression, Jesus is a refuge and strength for the oppressed (see Psalm 9:9). When we are feeling downcast, we can put our hope and trust in Jesus for he is our Savior and our God (see Psalm 42:5, 11). He upholds the cause of the oppressed, gives food to the hungry (see Psalm 146:5-7), and works righteousness and justice for them (see also Psalm 103:6). When our souls are downcast within us, we can remember God's promises and his faithful deeds. Because of his great love we are not consumed, for his compassions never fail. They are new and made available every morning (see Lamentations 3:19-23).

He lifts us out of the slimy pit, out of the mud and the mire. He sets our feet on a rock and gives us a firm place to stand. He puts a new song in our mouths, a song of praise (see Psalm 40:1-3). He keeps our lamp burning and turns darkness into light (see Psalm 18:28). He comforts us in our mourning, and provides for our grieving souls. He bestows on us a crown of beauty instead of ashes, the oil of gladness instead of mourning, and a garment of praise instead of a spirit of despair (see Isaiah 61:3). Whenever we are overwhelmed by life, he is our sanctuary and place of rest. He is our strength and our deliverer, the rock in whom we take refuge. He is our shield and salvation (see Psalm 18:1-2).

When the enemy of our souls tries to destroy us, God reaches down from on high and takes hold of us and draws us out of the deep waters. He rescues us from the enemy; from our foes who are too strong for us (see Psalm 18:16-17). When we dwell in the shelter of the Most High, we rest in the shadow of the Almighty. Under the protection of his wings, we are safe from the fowler's snare and the deadly pestilence. We need not fear, because he is our shield of protection (see Psalm 91:1-13).

When we do struggle with feelings of depression, we can turn to him and pray:

"To you, O LORD, I called; to the Lord I cried for mercy: What gain is there in my destruction, in my going down into the pit? Will the dust praise you? Will it proclaim your faithfulness? Hear, O LORD, and be merciful to me; O LORD, be my help" (Psalm 30:8-10). "Weeping may remain for a night, but rejoicing comes in the morning" (Psalm 30:5). In my pain I will remember all of your benefits—who forgives all my sins and heals all my diseases, who redeems my life from the pit, and crowns me with love and compassion; you are the One who satisfies my desires with good things (see Psalm 103:1-5).

"I will exalt you, O LORD, for you lifted me out of the depths and did not let my enemies gloat over me. O LORD my God, I called to you for help and you healed me. O LORD, you brought me up from the grave, you spared me from going down into the pit. You turned my wailing into dancing; you removed my sackcloth and clothed me with joy, that my heart may sing to you and not be silent. O LORD my God, I will give you thanks forever" (Psalm 30:1-3; 11-12).

Recommended Books and Resources

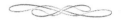

When treating depression, it is vital that the whole person—mind—body—spirit—be treated, not just the mind or emotional state. For more information about depression, treating depression, teens and depression, or ways to find hope and joy in the midst of depression, consider these books, or visit our website at www.LibertyinChristMinistries.com.

Experiencing Joy: Strategies for Living a Joy Filled Life, Patty Mason

The Power of Hope, Patty Mason

Hope Prevails: Insights from a Doctor's Personal Journey through Depression, Dr. Michelle Bengtson

Understanding and Loving a Person with Depression: Biblical and Practical Wisdom to Build Empathy, Preserve Boundaries, and Show Compassion, Stephen Arterburn, M.Ed. and Brenda Hunter, Ph.D.

218 Ways to Own Joy: An Interactive Journey Through All Bible Verses Containing 'Joy,' Lisa Miller-Rich

Honestly, Shelia Walsh

When the Darkness Will Not Lift: Doing What We Can While We Wait for God-and-Joy, John Piper

Get Out of that Pit: Straight Talk About God's Deliverance, Beth Moore

Acknowledgements

A very special thank you to all the precious souls who were willing to contribute to this book by sharing their testimonies of hardship and faith. May God bless you richly for your continued trust in him.

I want to extend a word of thanks to all the people who made a difference in my life. Terry Delong, Sue Jacox, Miriam Nodzo, Vivian Good, David Noel, and Fatima Eid, you are my mentors, the ones who stood with me through my personal journey, continually cheering me on toward the goal, and helping me remain focused on what is most important.

Thank you to my husband and family for their unwavering support. It's a scary thing to record your life on paper; it's even scarier to publish your life for others to read. This book was never meant to hurt those I love, air dirty laundry, or disparage anyone's character. Before publishing this book, I spoke with my husband and parents. All three have encouraged me to share my story. In many ways, sharing this book with my family brought us closer together and gave us a greater level of appreciation and respect for each other. I love my family dearly, and could not have openly shared some of the aspects of this book without their consent.

I want to thank my children for loving me unconditionally. They were very young at the time of the depression, yet the love they showed during that time was immeasurable and priceless. At times their love was the only thing that pulled me through some of those dark days. My children are amazing. I am proud of them; and, in spite of that terrible time, they have grown into wonderful adults.

I especially want to acknowledge my oldest daughter. While writing this book, we talked about her childhood and what happened during the depression. To my amazement, she only remembered two incidents. Unlike the first time I asked her to forgive me, she smiled warmly and hugged me as if to say *No apology was necessary*. But it was necessary—not only for her but for me. As we hugged, it reminded me of the incomparable joy of forgiveness and love.

Thank you to all the wonderful men and women who graciously took the time to review the manuscript and offer encouragement, advice, and recommendations. Your thoughts on this project are greatly appreciated. I couldn't have done this project without your support.

A special thank you to my editor, Peter Lundell, as well as Kristen Veldhuis, Dawn Staymates, and Bob Ousnamer at EA Books who helped with interior formatting and cover design to make this book a reality.

Finally, I want to acknowledge all the dear souls who approached me during this venture to share their hearts and hurts, struggles and pain. It was your stories that kept me on track, and inspired me to finish this book. I must admit, in moments of weakness, I wondered if what I was doing would make a difference in the lives of others. Many people are searching for answers, and at times I worried if my story would be enough. But as I listened to your stories, I would once again be reminded of the reason why I was writing this book. As I shared my story with you in return, I could see hope form in your eyes and would remember how my story points to Jesus. Jesus is enough. Jesus is the answer we all seek to find.

Therefore, to my loving Savior and Lord: Thank you for saving me. Thank you for being there in my darkest hour. Thank you for reaching into my well of depression, pulling me out and placing my life on the solid ground of your love. You, and you alone, broke the bonds of my depression without drugs. You are what I have searched for all my life—the answer to all my quests. You have filled my life with direction and purpose. You are my constant hope for today and tomorrow. You are the reason I have joy.

About the Author

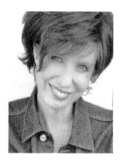

Patty Mason is a national speaker and the founder of Liberty in Christ Ministries. For more than two decades, Patty has shared her story of God's redeeming grace and deliverance from depression before numerous audiences, in several books, blogs, and magazines, such as Lifeway's "Living More," as well as radio and television programs, including American Family Radio, Moody Radio, and The 700 Club.

She has encouraged and challenged millions with God's word through Sisters on Assignment, Salem Communication's Light Source, and as the host of Joyful Living Radio. She has written several books and Bible Studies, including *Transformed by Desire*, *Experiencing Joy: Strategies for Living a Joy Filled Life*, and *The Power of Hope.*

Patty lives with her husband in Nashville, Tennessee.

To learn more about Patty, her books, or Liberty in Christ Ministries, visit:
www.LibertyinChristMinistries.com

[23] *Damaged Goods: Learning to Dream Again,* Charlotte Hunt, (Dream Madly Publishers: 2010)

[24] *A Scarlet Cord of Hope: My Journey through Guilt, Shame, and Fear to Hope,* Sheryl Griffin, (WordCraft Press, Nashville, TN: 2014).

Made in the USA
Coppell, TX
14 February 2020